# Interpreting Mu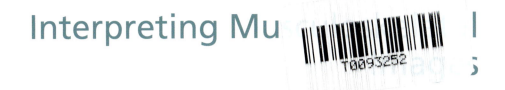

This visual manual is an accessible guide to musculoskeletal image interpretation and reporting, including common trauma pathologies, arthropathies, mechanisms of injury and classification systems. Beautifully illustrated with schematic line diagrams, supplemented with radiographs and scans, the content has been developed to enhance learning and understanding of both radiology and anatomy, and the relationship between them.

## Key features:

- Concise, yet highly informative
- Large, high-quality illustrations supplement and enhance the written descriptions, with colour-coding for rapid matching of image to corresponding text
- Relates imaging to underlying anatomy and pathology, aiding accurate interpretation
- Carefully designed to support rapid access in the clinical setting and ideal also as a revision aid during examination preparation

The book delivers hands-on support to junior doctors, other emergency medicine personnel and practising radiographers for use in the clinical setting and is also ideal for students preparing for qualifying examinations in medicine and radiography.

# Interpreting
# Musculoskeletal
# Images

## Anatomy, Pathology and Emergency Reporting

**Rosie Jones**

Advance Practice Radiographer
University Hospitals of North Midlands NHS Trust, UK

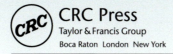

**CRC Press**
Taylor & Francis Group
Boca Raton  London  New York

CRC Press is an imprint of the
Taylor & Francis Group, an **informa** business

First edition published 2024
by CRC Press
6000 Broken Sound Parkway NW, Suite 300, Boca Raton, FL 33487-2742

and by CRC Press
4 Park Square, Milton Park, Abingdon, Oxon, OX14 4RN

*CRC Press is an imprint of Taylor & Francis Group, LLC*

© 2024 Rosie Jones

ISBN: 9781032409382 (hbk)
ISBN: 9781032398914 (pbk)
ISBN: 9781003355410 (ebk)

DOI: 10.1201/ 9781003355410

Typeset in Sabon
by Evolution Design & Digital

# Contents

# Acknowledgements

I would like to start by thanking the University Hospitals of North Midlands for their support in the publication of this book and for the use of Trust images in this publication. I would also like to thank my supportive colleagues within the UHNM Imaging Department and beyond for their support throughout, whether it has been assisting me in finding the images for publication or for helping with the ideas and concepts within the book itself.

Special thanks go to two people in particular; firstly, to Dr Anthony Taylor for taking time out of his busy schedule to read through the collection of notes that became this book and who added valuable suggestions that helped mould it into something that I never thought I would be able to produce.

And secondly, thanks must go to Dr Paul Hancock, without whom this book would not have seen the light of day. Your support throughout this process has been invaluable, and you have pushed me to produce something I never thought possible. Thank you for putting up with my constant silly questions and self-doubt; I could not have done this without your constant support and confidence in my abilities.

# About the Author

**Rosie Jones** is an Advanced Practice Radiographer specialising in musculoskeletal plain film image reporting. Since graduating from Birmingham City University in 2014, she began her career at the University Hospitals of North Midlands. Her experience working in a major trauma centre, combined with her passion for trauma imaging encouraged her to undertake a postgraduate qualification in musculoskeletal reporting at the University of Salford, graduating in 2021.

# Chapter 1

# Introduction

## Overview

This chapter will cover the structure of bones, joint anatomy and the different classifications of joints and their location within the body.

Starting at the microscopic level, anatomy and the difference between the range of cells which make up bone will be covered, followed by a basic introduction to bone formation, healing and the properties of bone and its ability to withstand and adapt to force.

An overview of fracture description will follow, introducing common fracture patterns and descriptions as well as an outline of the systematic approach of musculoskeletal X-ray review with a basic format for structured fracture description.

## Structure and properties of bones

### Bone cells

Bone is made up of four types of cells:

1. **Osteogenic cells:** stem cells found within the periosteum and bone marrow. Osteogenic cells are the only bone cells that can divide; they divide and differentiate into osteoblasts.
2. **Osteoblasts:** build bone. These are found in the parts of the bone responsible for growth such as the periosteum. The osteoblast produces collagen and calcium, which encase the osteoblast. Once fully encased, the osteoblast will mature resulting in the formation of an osteocyte.
3. **Osteocytes:** the primary cell of bone.
4. **Osteoclasts:** break bone down. Osteoclasts are large multi-nuclei cells which do not develop from osteogenic cells but develop from types of monocyte/macrophage cells. Osteoclasts work alongside osteoblasts to maintain healthy bone structure by removing old osteocytes, triggering the development and maturity of osteoblasts.

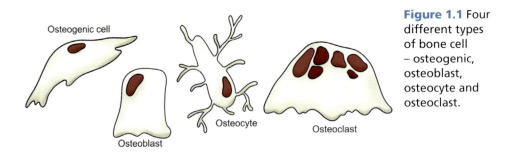

**Figure 1.1** Four different types of bone cell – osteogenic, osteoblast, osteocyte and osteoclast.

## Microscopic anatomy of bone

The most superficial layer of the bone is the periosteum; this is a layer of connective tissue containing blood vessels and nerves. Connecting the periosteum to the bone are strong collagen-based fibres called Sharpey's fibres.

The outer layer of the bone (or cortex) is made up of cortical bone. Cortical bone is made up of tightly packed, dense osteons which, in turn, are made up of concentric rings of bone cells called lamella surrounding the haversian canal. The Haversian canal contains the vascular and nervous supply to the bone. Between each osteon are Volkmann's canals, which assist with blood supply to the cortical bone.

The inner layer of bone is known as cancellous (trabecular/spongy) bone. This layer is not made up of osteons like cortical bones, cancellous bone has more of a honeycomb appearance made up of interconnected plates called trabeculae with the blood supply interwoven between the plates.

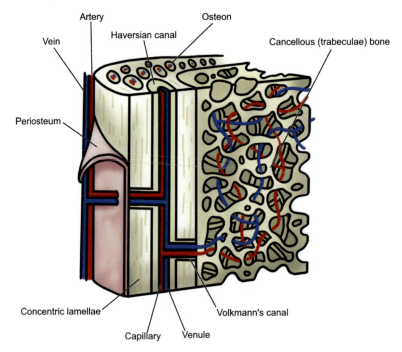

**Figure 1.2** Microscopic properties of bone.

## Bone development and growth

Bone development begins *in utero* and continues until the skeleton is fully developed in adulthood. Development begins when the fibrous membrane and hyaline cartilage that makes up a fetal skeleton begins to ossify. This is known as intramembranous ossification (development of bone from fibrous tissues) and endochondral ossification (development of bone from hyaline cartilage).

**Intramembranous ossification:** Seen in the development of flat bones, such as the bones of the skull and cranium. The fibrous membranes form a template which osteoblasts convert into bone by the secretion of collagen and calcium. This process converts the osteoblast into a mature osteocyte and ossifies the fibrous tissue.

**Endochondral ossification:** Seen in the development of the majority of bones in the body. The bones are primarily formed from hyaline cartilage which becomes encased in a membrane, called the perichondrium, containing blood vessels and osteoblasts (eventually the perichondrium will develop into the periosteum). The blood vessels help to distribute osteoblasts at the diaphysis of the bone which encase the diaphysis in a ring of cortical bone, whilst the cartilage in the centre of the diaphysis is replaced by cancellous bone, creating the primary ossification centre. This process continues within the diaphysis until osteoclasts begin to break down the centre of the cancellous bone in order to form the medullary cavity. The bone at the epiphysis develops in the same way. However, there is no osteoclast activity in the epiphysis, so the cancellous bone is not broken down and no medullary cavity is created. This creates the secondary ossification centres of the bone. A small layer of cartilage remains between the diaphysis and epiphysis forming the epiphyseal plate, which facilitates bone growth until skeletal maturity.

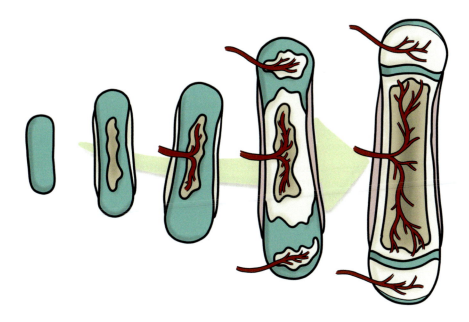

**Figure 1.3** Different stages of endochondral ossification.

## Types of bone

Different types of bone can be classified in several different ways. The first classification can be the axial and appendicular skeleton:

- **Axial:** Skull and face, spine, thorax, and sternum
- **Appendicular:** Limbs, hands, feet, shoulder girdle, pelvis.

Bones can also be further divided by shape:

- **Flat bones:** Skull, sternum
- **Long bones:** Humerus, radius/ulna, femur, tibia/fibula
- **Irregular bones:** Vertebra
- **Short bones:** Carpal and tarsal bones
- **Sesamoid bone:** Patella.

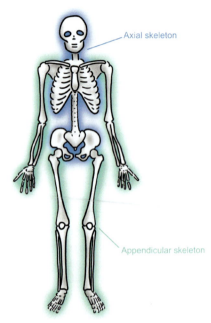

Axial skeleton

Appendicular skeleton

**Figure 1.4** Outline of the axial and appendicular skeleton.

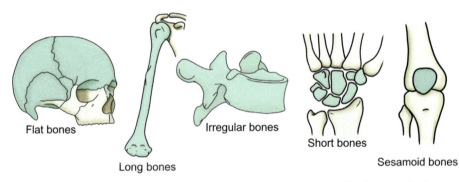

Flat bones

Long bones

Irregular bones

Short bones

Sesamoid bones

**Figure 1.5** Different types of bone within the human skeleton – flat bones (skull vault), long bones (humerus), irregular bones (vertebra), short bones (carpal bones) and sesamoid bones (patella).

## Anisotropic properties of bone

The bones' ability to withstand force. Bones are strongest in the longitudinal axis and weakest in its transverse axis, with varying strengths of force through the oblique angles.

This is due to the structure of bones, the osteons that make up bone are cylindrical and therefore withstand strong longitudinal forces. For example, try squashing a toilet roll along its longitudinal axis, it's very hard to do. But if you apply pressure to the middle of the roll it will collapse with a lot less force. It is the same principle.

## Viscoelastic properties of bone

The bones' ability to respond to force (different tissues have different viscoelastic properties).

Up to a certain point (the yield point), force can be applied to a bone and, once this force is removed, the bone will return to its normal state with no lasting damage. If the level of force surpasses the yield point, the bone will be unable to return to its normal state. If this force continues, the bone will reach its failure point, which is the point when a fracture occurs.

In trauma situations, the force applied to the bone is usually high and happens quickly; the bone reaches its failure point quickly and fractures occur.

## Wolff's law

Healthy bone has an ability to adapt to the demands and stresses placed upon it. The bone elements will place themselves in the direction of functional forces and can increase or decrease the bones' mass in response to the level of force. This can be seen as an increase in trabecular within bone (typically seen in the hip) or in a loss of bony density (seen in osteopenia e.g. disuse osteopenia). This can also be seen in degenerative processes such as osteoarthritis, as the articular surface wears down, the body recognises that the joint is unable to resist force and increases bone density (increased sclerosis) and increases surface area (osteophyte formation).

# Structure and types of joints

A joint is an articulation between two bones supported by ligaments. There are several different categories of joint with different joint types allowing for different movement.

Joint movement can be classified in three different ways:

1. **Synarthroses:** Immobile joint
2. **Amphiarthrosis:** Partial movement
3. **Diarthrosis:** Free moving joint.

As well as description of movement, joints can be categorised by their structure. The three main joint classifications are:

1. Fibrous joints
2. Cartilaginous joints
3. Synovial joints.

## Fibrous joints

This type of joint has no joint cavity containing fluid with the connection between the two articulating bones made through connective tissue.

Examples include:

- **Suture joint:** Found in the skull connecting the cranial bones. This joint is synarthrotic.
- **Gomphosis:** The only example of this joint is the joint of the teeth into the mandible. This joint is synarthrotic (in healthy adults).
- **Syndesmosis joint:** A fibrous joint made up of ligaments, examples can be found between tibia and fibula as well as the radius and ulna. This joint is amphiarthrotic.

## Cartilaginous joints

Like the fibrous joint, there is no joint cavity containing fluid connected with cartilage. The articulation between the two bones is made using hyaline cartilage or fibrocartilage.

There are two main types:

- **Synchondroses:** This is cartilage within bone, such as the epiphyseal plate in growing bone. This joint is synarthrotic.
- **Symphyses:** This is a fibrocartilaginous connection between two bones. Examples include the joint connecting the ribs to the sternum, the connection of the pubic bones (pubic symphyses) and the joint between the vertebral bodies, with the intervertebral disc acting as a fibrocartilaginous joint. These joints are amphiarthrotic.

## Synovial joints

Synovial joints are made up of a joint cavity containing synovial fluid. All synovial joints are diarthrotic and allow for a range of different movements.

The two articulating bones are lines with cartilage at the joint (hyaline cartilage). This cartilage helps reduce friction when the joint is moving. The joints are surrounded by the synovial capsule made up of a fibrous layer encasing the joint and holding it in shape, and a synovial membrane which produces the synovial fluid.

Synovial fluid builds up within the capsule and further helps to reduce friction when the joint is moving. The fluid also plays a role in reducing the effect of impacting forces on the joint and helps to regulate nutrition within the joint.

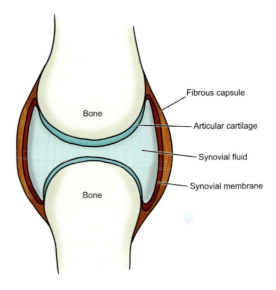

**Figure 1.6** The major components of a synovial joint.

## *Types of synovial joint*

There are six main types of synovial joint, all of which are diarthrotic. However, not all synovial joints have a full range of movement. Movement can be described as uniaxial (one plane of movement), biaxial (two planes of movement) or multiaxial (more than two planes of movement).

The six types of synovial joint are:

Plane joint: A uniaxial joint made up of two flat bone surfaces articulating. Examples include the intercarpal and intertarsal joint, the facet joints of the spine and the acromioclavicular joints.

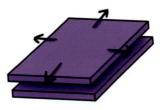

**Figure 1.7** A plane joint.

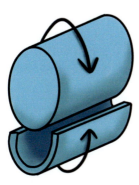

Hinge joint: A uniaxial which acts like a hinge of a door. One of the articulating surfaces has a concave appearance which sits within its corresponding convex surface of the second bone. Examples include elbow and knee joints.

**Figure 1.8** A hinge joint.

Pivot joint: A uniaxial joint which allows rotational movement in one axis. Examples include the atlantoaxial joint of C1/C2.

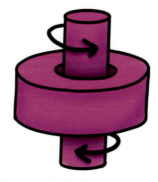

**Figure 1.9** A pivot joint.

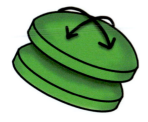

Condylar joint: A biaxial joint. One side of the joint has a convex ellipsoid appearance communicating with the other concave surface. These joints allow several different movements such as flexion/extension, abduction/adduction and circumduction. The appearance is similar to a ball and socket joint; however, they are not as deep or free moving. Examples include the 2nd–5th metacarpophalangeal joints.

**Figure 1.10** A condylar joint.

Saddle joint: A biaxial joint. The articular surface of both aspects of the joints has a concave and convex appearance and look like two saddles interlocked. Examples include the first carpometacarpal joints and the sternoclavicular joints.

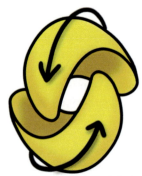

**Figure 1.11** A saddle joint.

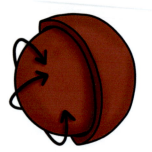

Ball & socket joint: A multiaxial joint. The articular surface of one bone sits within the concave, cup-like depression of the other bone. Allows for movement in all planes – flexion/extension, abduction/adduction, circumduction and rotation. Examples include the glenohumeral joints and the hip joints.

**Figure 1.12** A ball and socket joint.

# Describing fractures

There are many ways of describing fractures and developing a systematic approach to this helps to make the description process easier.

The first thing to describe is what type of fracture is present. There are many different fracture types, and they can be classified in several different ways. Firstly, is the fracture complete or incomplete? Complete fractures extend across the entirety of the bone breaking both cortices, for example, a transverse or oblique fracture. Incomplete fractures will not damage the entire cortex and predominantly occur in paediatric patients. Examples include the greenstick fracture or cortical bowing.

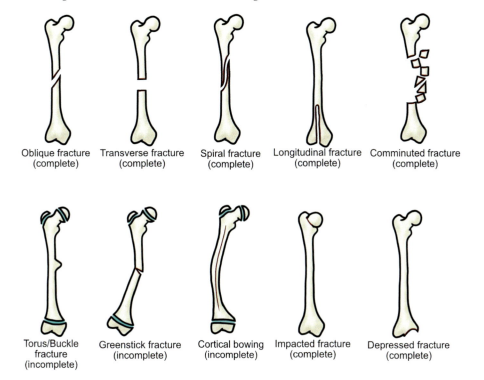

Oblique fracture (complete)  Transverse fracture (complete)  Spiral fracture (complete)  Longitudinal fracture (complete)  Comminuted fracture (complete)

Torus/Buckle fracture (incomplete)  Greenstick fracture (incomplete)  Cortical bowing (incomplete)  Impacted fracture (complete)  Depressed fracture (complete)

**Figure 1.13** Different types of fractures, covering both complete and incomplete fracture patterns.

The next thing to describe is where the fracture has occurred. Describe which bone/bones are involved and which part of the bone has been damaged.

Long bones can be described using three regions:

1. **Diaphysis**: The shaft of the bone.
2. **Metaphysis**: The point at which the bone becomes wider adjacent to the growth plate.
3. **Epiphysis**: The end of the bone adjacent to the joint.

In some cases, certain bones have similar descriptive terms for their anatomical regions, such as the head, neck and shaft of the metacarpals/metatarsals and the waist and poles of the scaphoid.

It is also important to identify if the fracture involves a joint surface (intra-articular). Intra-articular fractures sometimes require different treatment and are at a higher risk of future complications such as secondary osteoarthritis.

The final thing to describe is the displacement or movement of the fracture.

Using the anatomical position, describe the movement of the distal part of the fracture fragment in relation to the proximal part. The displacement of the fracture can be in one plane, or have multiple planes of movement, and can include full displacement, angulation/tilt, impaction/bony override, distraction/diastasis, or rotation.

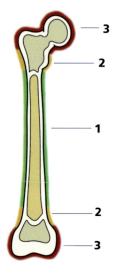

**Figure 1.14** Illustration highlighting the different anatomical regions of a long bone.

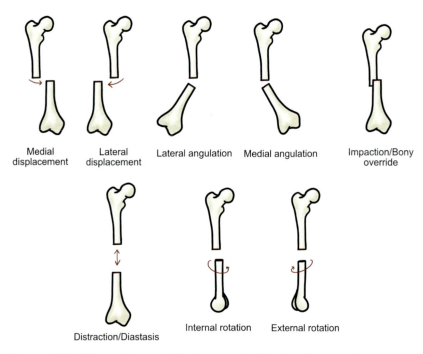

**Figure 1.15** Different types of displacement of fracture fragments.

# Bone healing

The process of bone healing usually takes place over four stages:

1. **Inflammation (week 1):**  Fracture causes the formation of a haematoma and inflammation. Granulation tissue is formed (new connective and vascular tissues). This is the stage in which the patient may experience pain, swelling and possibly crepitus at the fracture site.
2. **Soft callus (weeks 2–3):** The fractured bone ends begin to 'die back' with the osteoclasts removing the dead bone tissue. The granulation tissue is replaced with fibrous tissues and cartilage. In some cases, fractures that were previously occult may be visible at this stage e.g. non-displaced scaphoid fractures.
3. **Hard callus (weeks 4–12):** Osteoblast bone formation begins. Calcium is laid down, forming a callus that can be seen on X-ray, the fracture site becomes more stable and rigid, and crepitus is reduced significantly.
4. **Remodelling (months +):** Lamellar bone is laid down and normal bone density is restored. In children, the bone usually completely remodels with the hard callus shrinking and the bone contours returning to normal (on follow-up X-ray, it may be difficult to see if a fracture ever occurred). In adults, this process is rarely fully completed and there is usually some evidence of previous fractures (bony remodelling).

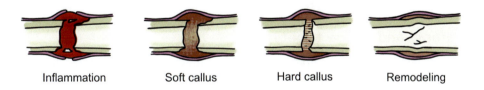

Inflammation          Soft callus          Hard callus          Remodeling

**Figure 1.16** The four stages of bone healing: inflammation, soft callus formation, hard callus formation and remodelling.

# AABCS of musculoskeletal image interpretation

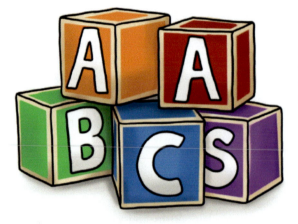

## AABCS

- Anatomy and image quality
- Alignment
- Bones
- Cartilage
- Soft tissues

**Figure 1.17** AABCS building blocks.

Before beginning to evaluate an image always check it is the correct patient!

Check the date and time stamp on the image (don't diagnose an old film) and check to see if the patient has any previous imaging for comparison.

## Anatomy and image quality

Check the image produced is appropriate to answer the clinical question. Will your request allow this to be demonstrated? This is where the clinical information provided to the radiographer is important; give as much information as possible – explain the mechanism of injury and clinical presentation (if there is tenderness, bruising, swelling etc. where it is). For example, 'FOOSH injury to right hand, swelling over wrist, bony tenderness distal radius. ?fracture'. Radiographers are independent practitioners and will produce the images suitable to the request, which may include additional supplementary views to assist with diagnosis.

Is the image produced diagnostic? Can you see all the required anatomy (including soft tissues)? Can you assess the bony trabecula pattern? Is there any rotation or poor positioning which may obscure pathology?

**Develop pattern recognition:** Knowing what normal looks like is key; understanding the position of bony tuberosities, accessory ossicles, normal variants, etc. Understand the differences between the mature and immature skeleton.

## Alignment

This brings the focus to the joint (be aware of what type of joint you are assessing), not just for the assessment of the bony component, but also to assess the articular surface, fibrous regions, ligament and tendon attachments.

Evaluation:

- Is the joint space equidistant and within normal range for that joint e.g. carpal joints = 2 mm.
- Do the bones on either side of the joint align? Assess this by drawing a line down the centre and sides of the bone to assess for alignment. This line should not jump or have any significant steps.

## Bones

Understand the appearance of normal bone.

Be systematic in your approach:

1. **Trace the cortex of each bone individually**: Check for steps, breaks, angulation and periosteal reaction.
2. **Internal structure**: Check the trabecular pattern for gaps or irregularity.
3. **Scan the entire image:** Step back and look for irregularities – lucent or sclerotic regions will stand out.

Be aware of normal variants such as nutrient channels (arterial channels for the primary ossification centre, as the bone grows, they elongate in the direction of the bone growth and should have a well corticated edge), clefts, accessory ossicles, etc.

## Cartilage

Healthy cartilage should be radiolucent and not visible on X-ray; however it is still important to check the space it occupies.

Check for opacity within the joint space. This may be caused by long-standing changes such as chondrocalcinosis (build-up of calcium pyrophosphate crystals in the joint – linked to arthropathy) or calcification of soft-tissue structures, or by acute injury such as subchondral fractures or loose body within the joint.

## Soft tissues

Soft tissues should be seen on X-ray as a range of different shades of grey. Under- or over-exposure of the X-ray can obliterate the soft tissues and prevent true visualisation.

Fat is important! It outlines the structures, movement of fat pads or fat planes and can indicate acute injury or pathology

Evaluation:

- Soft tissue should follow the bone contours.
- Be aware of normal soft-tissue depths. Swelling can indicate site of acute injury and regions with tissue swelling should always be thoroughly assessed.
- Be aware of normal structures, such as sesamoid bones, which appear within the soft tissues.

# Chapter 2

# Upper Limb

## Overview

This chapter will cover the review of the upper limb including the shoulder girdle, elbow, forearm and hand.

An initial review of upper limb anatomy will be followed by an introduction to common trauma and radiographic appearance of trauma within each anatomical region of the upper limb. An introduction to regional systematic reviews will follow using a concise revision format.

## Anatomy

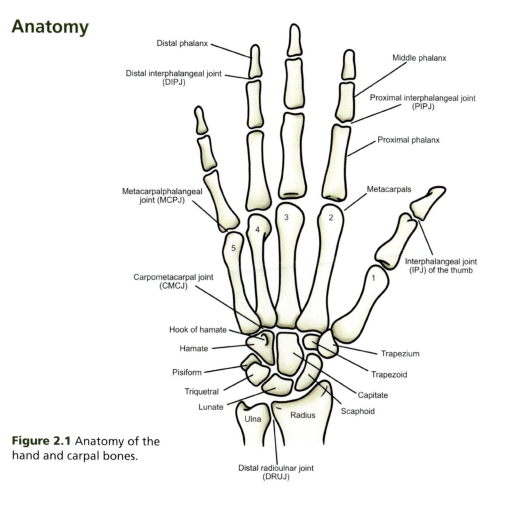

**Figure 2.1** Anatomy of the hand and carpal bones.

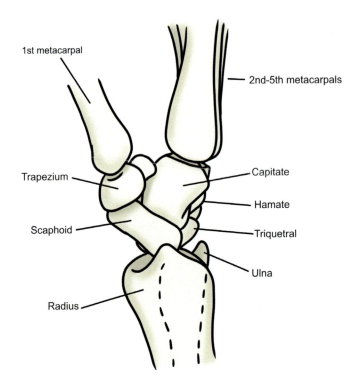

**Figure 2.2** Anatomy of the lateral carpal region.

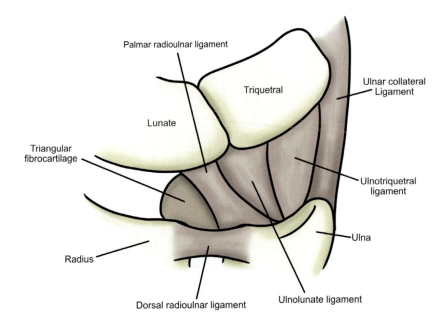

**Figure 2.3** Anatomy of the triangular fibrocartilage complex (TFCC).

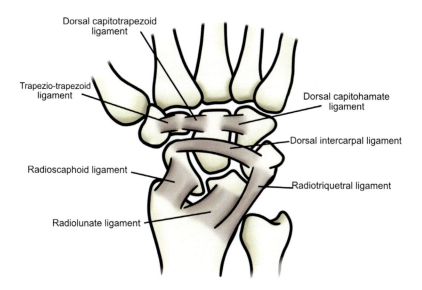

**Figure 2.4** Anatomy of the carpal ligaments – palmer aspect.

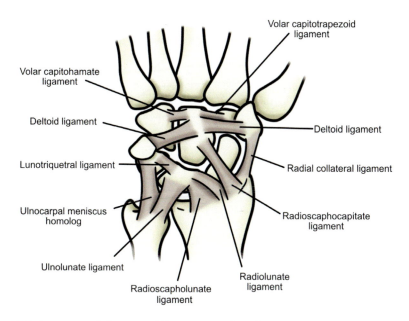

**Figure 2.5** Anatomy of the carpal ligaments – dorsal aspect.

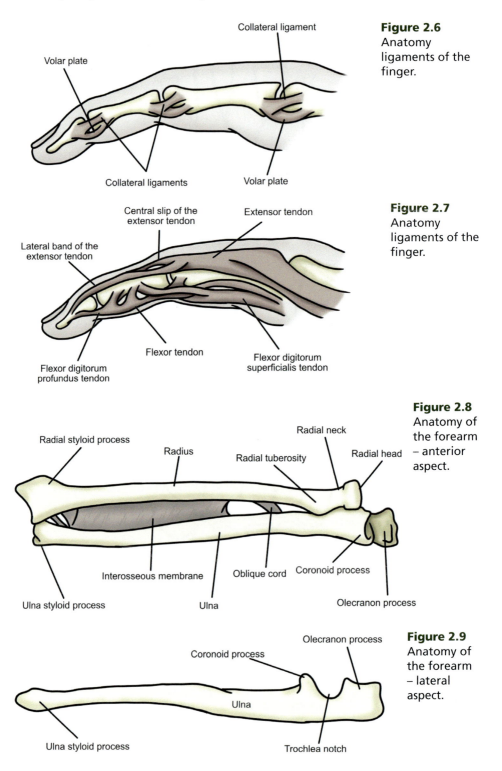

Collateral ligament

Volar plate

Collateral ligaments

Volar plate

**Figure 2.6**
Anatomy
ligaments of the
finger.

Central slip of the
extensor tendon

Extensor tendon

Lateral band of the
extensor tendon

Flexor tendon

Flexor digitorum
profundus tendon

Flexor digitorum
superficialis tendon

**Figure 2.7**
Anatomy
ligaments of the
finger.

Radial styloid process

Radius

Radial neck

Radial tuberosity

Radial head

Interosseous membrane

Oblique cord

Coronoid process

Ulna styloid process

Ulna

Olecranon process

**Figure 2.8**
Anatomy of
the forearm
– anterior
aspect.

Olecranon process

Coronoid process

Ulna

Ulna styloid process

Trochlea notch

**Figure 2.9**
Anatomy of
the forearm
– lateral
aspect.

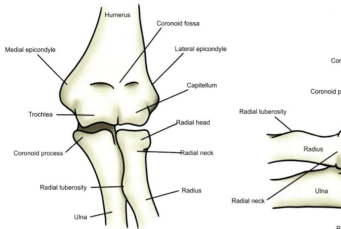

**Figure 2.10** Anatomy of the Elbow – anterior aspect.

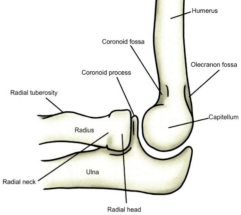

**Figure 2.11** Anatomy of the elbow – lateral aspect.

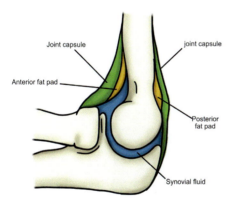

**Figure 2.12** Anatomy of the elbow capsule – lateral aspect.

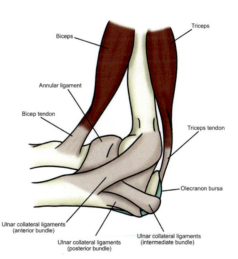

**Figure 2.13** Anatomy of the ligaments of the elbow joint.

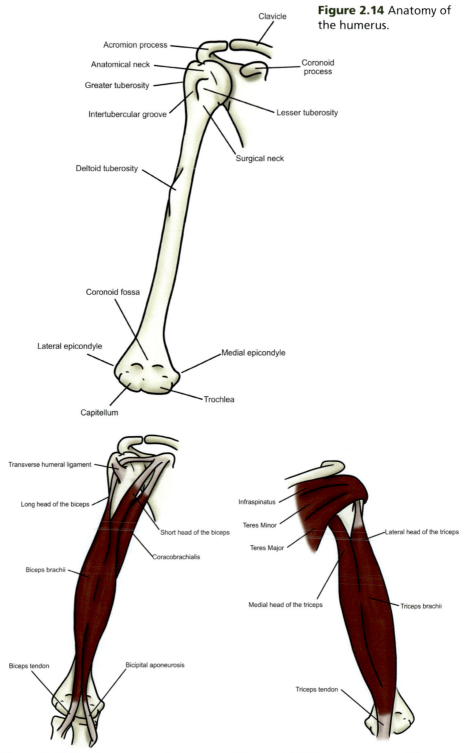

**Figure 2.14** Anatomy of the humerus.

Clavicle

Acromion process

Anatomical neck

Greater tuberosity

Intertubercular groove

Coronoid process

Lesser tuberosity

Surgical neck

Deltoid tuberosity

Coronoid fossa

Lateral epicondyle

Medial epicondyle

Trochlea

Capitellum

Transverse humeral ligament

Long head of the biceps

Short head of the biceps

Coracobrachialis

Biceps brachii

Biceps tendon

Bicipital aponeurosis

Infraspinatus

Teres Minor

Teres Major

Lateral head of the triceps

Medial head of the triceps

Triceps brachii

Triceps tendon

**Figure 2.15** Muscle anatomy of the upper arm – anterior aspect.

**Figure 2.16** Muscle anatomy of the upper arm – posterior aspect.

# Hand Trauma

Phalangeal fractures are relatively common. Mechanisms which commonly cause fracture and injury to the phalanges include crushing, twisting forces and avulsion force (such as hyperextension or hyperflexion). Avulsion injuries (particularly involving the fingers) are easily missed; however, detection of these injuries is important as the fingers are functionally important and small fractures can have a huge impact as fingers are so important to the activities of daily life. Small fractures can impact upon work, life or hobbies.

> **TIP**
>
> 'Small' injuries to fingers are easily missed, but have a big impact. Examine thoroughly.

## Distal phalanx

Fractures of the distal phalanx (DP) typically result from crush injury and are usually related to a sports or work injury. DP fractures account for more than 50% of all DP fractures and usually involve the terminal tuft. Patients typically present with tenderness, swelling, deformity and/or crepitus. Open wounds (usually involving the nail bed) are commonly associated with fractures of the distal phalanx and are at risk of contamination and infection, which will then impact upon healing. Closed fractures are considered stable, especially when the fracture is extra-articular. Fractures involving the base of the phalanx are often unstable as this is the region where the flexor and extensor tendons insert.

Fracture types include:

- Vertical split fractures.
- **Shaft fractures:** Tend to be vertical or transverse with angulation, which can be demonstrated on the lateral X-ray.
- **Crush fractures:** These are common (usually involving the terminal tuft).
- **Mallet finger deformity.**

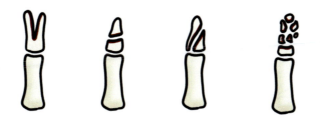

**Figure 2.17** Different types of distal phalangeal fractures commonly seen in the fingers – vertical fractures, fractures involving the shaft and comminuted fractures.

### Middle phalanx

The middle phalanx is the least commonly fractured phalanx. Fractures here usually occur following a hyperextension mechanism, resulting in a volar plate fracture. These fractures are avulsion fractures at the insertion point of the volar plate and the fracture fragment is often very small and can be difficult to identify. True lateral or oblique imaging is needed in order to demonstrate small fragments and associated soft-tissue swelling can indicate fracture.

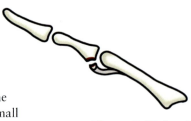

**Figure 2.18** A volar plate fracture.

### Proximal phalanx

The proximal phalanx is the most common phalanx fracture seen in paediatric patients. Fractures tend to be spiral or transverse and the digit is often shortened and rotated. The rotational deformity is more obvious when the patient's fingers are flexed. Fracture angulation is best demonstrated on the lateral or oblique X-ray with the DP view usually underestimating the fracture angulation.

> ### TIP
>
> Asking patients to flex fingers during clinical examination will make a rotational deformity more prominent.

### Mallet finger deformity

This usually results from a direct blow to an extended finger or a laceration to the dorsal aspect of the distal interphalangeal joint (DIPJ). This causes a rupture of the extensor tendon or an avulsion fracture at the insertion point of the tendon at the base of the distal phalanx. However, an avulsion fracture is less commonly seen. Patients present with swelling and tenderness (especially along the DIPJ) with the fingertip flexed at 45° with an inability to straighten. It is important for the imaging of Mallet finger deformities to be performed without the use of radiographic positioning aids (such as positioning supports or immobilisation aids) as these will support the finger in extension and mask the true extent of the Mallet finger deformity.

**Figure 2.19** Mallet finger deformity.

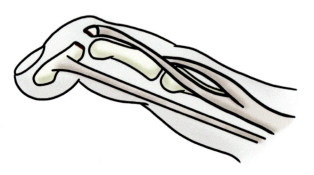

## Boutonnière deformity

This deformity can result from forced flexion of the proximal interphalangeal joint (PIPJ) or from a laceration to the dorsal aspect of the finger. It is also a deformity commonly seen in rheumatoid arthritis (RA). Injury causes a rupture of the central slip of the extensor ligament with associated migration of the lateral bands downwards. This results in extension of the PIPJ with flexion at the DIPJ.

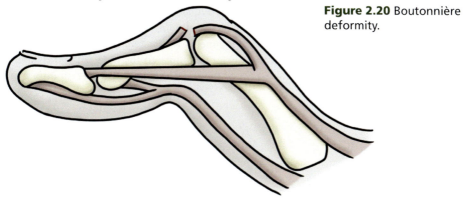

**Figure 2.20** Boutonnière deformity.

## Metacarpal fractures

Fractures of the metacarpals are a very commonly seen injury following trauma to the hand. These fractures are seen as a result of a direct blow to the hand or axial loading, such as punch-like injuries, hyperextension or a high-energy mechanism such as a road traffic collision. Patients will present with variable amounts of soft-tissue swelling, tenderness, deformity (such as rotation or foreshortening) and wounds in the region of injury, which may indicate an open fracture. Motor deficit is rarely seen in metacarpal fractures unless there has been associated tendon damage.

Fractures can be described according to the anatomical region of the metacarpal affecting the head, neck, shaft, or base. Fractures of the neck and shaft of the metacarpal are often associated with punch-like mechanisms involving axial loading into a clenched fist and are commonly seen at the fifth metacarpal (boxer's fracture) with associated palmar angulation of the distal fracture fragments. Although commonly seen at the fifth metacarpal, boxer-type fractures can be seen at other metacarpals.

Further fractures include oblique fractures involving the metacarpal shaft or base. If the fracture occurs at the base of the metacarpal, there may be associated carpometacarpal joint (CMCJ) dislocation or subluxation. After the fifth metacarpal, the first metacarpal is the second most commonly fractured metacarpal, with fractures usually involving the base of the first metacarpal (78%).

Fractures commonly seen at the first metacarpal include:

● **Bennett's fracture:** An oblique intra-articular fracture at the base of the first metacarpal with dorsal subluxation or dislocation of the first CMCJ joint. Fracture displacement is worsened by the abductor muscle of the first metacarpal. Typically seen following axial loading with the thumb in extension, such as in a fall or punch-like mechanism. Patients will present with swelling, tenderness (particularly at the CMCJ), bruising and reduced range of movement.

- **Rolando fracture:** Similar to a Bennett's fracture. However, the fracture is comminuted and intra-articular, with the fracture pattern appearing in a T or Y shape. Typically seen following axial loading with the thumb in extension, such as in a fall or punch-like mechanism. Patients will present with swelling, tenderness (particularly at the CMCJ), bruising and reduced range of movement.
- **Gamekeepers/Skiers thumb:** Caused by hyperabduction of the first metacarpal phalangeal joint (MCPJ) with outward distraction of the thumb. This causes the ulna collateral ligament to rupture or causes an avulsion fracture at the insertion point of the ligament. Patients present with swelling and pain. Location of the pain can give an indication to which of the collateral ligaments is affected: if the pain is at the ulna/medial aspect of the thumb this can indicate an injury to the ulna collateral ligament; if the pain is at the radial/lateral aspect of the thumb this can indicate an injury to the radial collateral ligament.

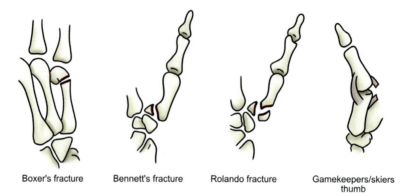

Boxer's fracture    Bennett's fracture    Rolando fracture    Gamekeepers/skiers thumb

**Figure 2.21** Four types of fractures and soft-tissue injuries seen within the metacarpals; boxers' fractures, involving the neck of the 5th metacarpal, Bennett's and Rolando fractures, involving the base of the 1st metacarpal and Gamekeepers/Skiers thumb, a ligamentous injury involving the MCPJ of the thumb.

## Carpometacarpal dislocations

Carpometacarpal dislocations are rare, accounting for less than 1% of all hand and wrist injuries and are associated with high-energy mechanisms of injury involving axial loading or direct blow to the carpometacarpal region. Patients will present with pain and significant swelling, which can be localised to the specific joint affected. If the dislocation is affecting the fifth CMCJ, there may be deviation of the fifth finger. However, dependent upon the amount of swelling present, this deformity may be masked.

The fifth CMCJ is the most commonly seen dislocated CMCJ accounting for 50% of CMCJ dislocations and is usually associated with further dislocation of another CMCJ. The majority of CMCJ malalignments involve dorsal dislocation (66%) and can be easily missed due to overlapping anatomy within the carpal region.

Check for loss of alignment. The CMCJ should demonstrate clear joint spaces with a typical zig-zag pattern of the CMCJ on the DP view (blue line). Loss of normal alignment can be more obvious on the lateral or oblique X-rays.

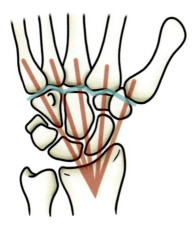

**Figure 2.22** Normal alignment of the carpometacarpal joints.

## Carpal arcs

The carpal joint spaces should be uniform and parallel, measuring approximately 1–2 mm (in adults). The carpal arcs (also known as Gilula arcs) are three lines used to assess the carpal alignment on the DP X-ray. Each line should be smooth and continuous with no steps or breaks.

Arc 1: Runs from the proximal aspect of the scaphoid, along the proximal aspect of the lunate and finally the proximal triquetral.

Arc 2: Runs from the distal aspect of the scaphoid, along the distal aspect of the lunate and finally the distal triquetral.

Arc 3: Runs around the proximal aspect of the capitate and proximal aspect of the hamate.

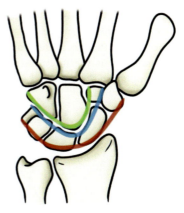

**Figure 2.23** Normal appearance and alignment of the carpal arcs.

## Carpal zone of vulnerability

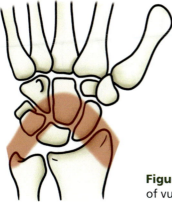

This is the region of the carpus where most fractures or dislocations occur. As you progress from the radial to the ulna aspect, the severity of injury increases. However, the frequency of this injury occurring decreases.

For example, a radial styloid fracture is considered a common injury in this region. However, it is usually not a severe injury. A fracture of the ulna styloid process is less commonly seen and is usually related to more severe injury.

**Figure 2.24** The position of the carpal zone of vulnerability.

## Scaphoid fractures

Fractures of the scaphoid tend to occur following axial loading onto a hyperextended wrist and are commonly seen after a fall onto outstretched hand (FOOSH), road traffic collision or sporting injury. Patients present with varying amounts of pain, tenderness over the anatomical snuff box (ASB) or in the region of the scaphoid tubercle or focal swelling. Pain and tenderness may be more apparent when axial force is applied to the thumb metacarpal, which can be assessed clinically using the scaphoid compression test. Bruising is not commonly seen in acute scaphoid injury.

Most scaphoid fractures are un-displaced fractures involving the waist of the scaphoid. These can be difficult to identify or occult on initial X-ray imaging. If there is clinical suspicion for an un-displaced scaphoid fracture treatment (splinting) follow-up imaging, usually 10–14 days post injury, should be considered. As the scaphoid begins to heal, there will be reabsorption of the bone and increased sclerosis, at which point, the previously occult fracture will be visible on X-ray.

Fractures of the distal pole of the scaphoid are usually associated with avulsion involving the radial collateral ligament. These fractures tend to heal quickly as the distal pole of the scaphoid has its own blood supply. The blood supply to the proximal pole of the scaphoid enters in the region of the waist. As a fracture to the waist of the scaphoid disrupts the blood supply, there is an increased risk of fracture non-union or avascular necrosis. This risk increases as the fractures move closer to the proximal pole of the scaphoid as the blood supply to the scaphoid only comes from this one direction.

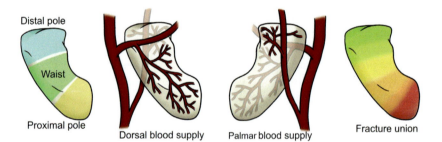

**Figure 2.25** The bony and vascular anatomy of the scaphoid and a representation of the rates of fracture union in the scaphoid, showing good union rates at the distal pole, with non-union seen more commonly at the proximal pole.

## Scapholunate interval

The scapholunate interval is a radiographic measurement taken on the DP image. In adults, this joint space is usually approximately 2 mm. In paediatric patients, the joint space appears wider due to the cartilaginous components of the carpus.

Widening of the joint space can indicate injury of the scapholunate ligament and is diagnostic of scapholunate dislocation.

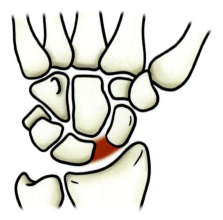

**Figure 2.26** Illustration demonstrating widening of the scapholunate interval indicating ligamentous injury.

## Carpal dislocations

Dislocations involving the carpal region are uncommon, with most true dislocations involving the lunate. Fractures with associated dislocations are more commonly seen and usually occur within the carpal zone of vulnerability. These injuries are a result of loading onto an extended or ulnar deviated hand and are associated with high-energy mechanisms such as a fall from height or road traffic collision. Patients will present with pain and swelling with significant pain when the patient attempts to extend the fingers. As a result, the patient will prefer to hold their hand with the fingers in flexion.

When assessing for dislocations/fracture-dislocations, it is important to assess the relationship of the lunate and the other carpal bones on the lateral X-ray. The lunate should articulate with the radius proximally and the capitate distally. The convex aspect of the lunate should face upwards with the capitate sitting within it.

- **Lunate dislocation:** On lateral X-ray, the lunate appears to slip forwards to the palmar (anterior) aspect, with the concave surface tilting anteriorly and empty. On DP X-ray, the lunate looks triangular and the joint spaces, particularly the scapholunate joint, appear widened.
- **Peri-lunate dislocation:** Less common than the lunate dislocation and usually associated with other injury. On lateral X-ray, the lunate stays in its normal position with the capitate and metacarpals dorsally displaced (but still aligned with each other).
- **Mid-carpal dislocation:** The lunate tilts anteriorly and subluxes from the radius, with an associated dorsal dislocation of the capitate from the lunate. However, the dislocation isn't usually as severe as it is in a true peri-lunate dislocation.

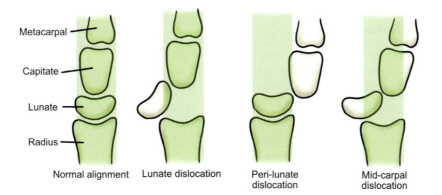

Metacarpal

Capitate

Lunate

Radius

Normal alignment   Lunate dislocation   Peri-lunate dislocation   Mid-carpal dislocation

**Figure 2.27** Normal alignment of the carpal region on lateral X-ray and the three main types of carpal dislocation – a lunate dislocation, peri-lunate dislocation and a mid-carpal dislocation.

## Triquetral fracture

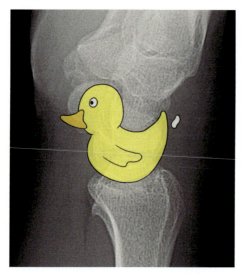

**Figure 2.28** Image demonstrating the 'pooping duck sign' as seen on lateral wrist X-ray with a triquetral fracture. © 2022 University Hospitals of North Midlands NHS Trust. All rights reserved.

This is the second most commonly fractured carpal bone. Commonly caused by a FOOSH with dorsiflexion and ulnar deviation of the wrist. This causes the ulna styloid process to impact on the triquetral and 'chips' away a fleck of bone. This bone fragment is demonstrated on the lateral projection with associated soft-tissue swelling – 'pooping duck' sign. Other mechanisms of injury include hyperflexion of the wrist joint; this causes strain on the dorsal ligaments and results in an avulsion type fracture.

Patients present with swelling, particularly at the dorsal aspect of the dorsal and medial aspect of the hand with pain at the triquetral and when flexing or extending the wrist or hand.

## Kienböck disease

Avascular necrosis of the lunate which can result from a single or repeated trauma or dislocation of the lunate (causing disruption to the lunate's blood supply). Once necrosis begins, there is an established progression/appearance of the lunate.

- **Stage 1:** Fracture of the lunate – no visible changes on X-ray, indistinguishable from a wrist sprain.
- **Stage 2:** Increased sclerosis of the lunate.
- **Stage 3a:** Flattening of the lunate.
- **Stage 3b:** Flattening/collapse of the lunate with fixed rotation of the scaphoid. Stages 3a and 3b may also demonstrate proximal migration of the capitate.
- **Stage 4:** Almost complete collapse of the lunate with associated degenerative changes seen within the carpus, including joint space narrowing, osteophyte formation, sclerosis and degenerative cyst formation.

Treatment and management changes with the progression of the disease. Stage 1 can be treated with immobilisation and support. Stages 2 and 3a usually require surgery (such as revascularisation procedures or joint levelling procedures), late stages (Stages 3b or Stage 4) can indicate complete fusion surgery or carpectomy are required.

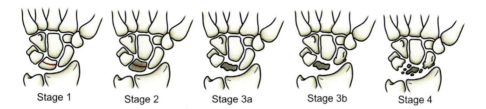

Stage 1          Stage 2          Stage 3a          Stage 3b          Stage 4

**Figure 2.29** The five stages of Kienböck disease.

# Wrist Trauma

The most common mechanism of injury of the wrist is a fall onto outstretched hand (FOOSH). This mechanism tends to cause specific injury patterns dependent on the patient's age.

- **4–10 years:** Torus type fracture of the distal radius
- **11–16 years:** Salter-Harris type II fracture
- **17–40 years:** Scaphoid fracture
- **Over 40 years:** Colles' type fracture.

## Normal anatomy and alignment

**PA X-ray:** The distal radial articular surface tilts anteriorly 17° towards the ulna with the medial aspect of the radius articulating with the ulna notch. The ulna should appear marginally shorter than the radius. The distal radius in adult patients may demonstrate a subtle sclerotic line. However, this is the epiphyseal scar and should not be confused with a fracture. The carpal arcs should remain uniform throughout.

Lateral X-ray: The distal articular surface should be angled approximately 10°–15° anteriorly (subtle fractures can flatten this angle). The articular surfaces of the radius, lunate and capitate should remain congruent and aligned.

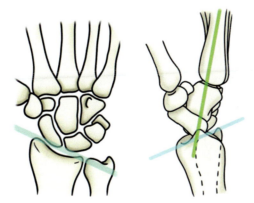

**Figure 2.30** Normal alignment and angles of the distal radius, ulna, and carpal region.

## Pronator quadratus fat pad

This is seen as a dark line within the anterior soft tissues at the distal radius, visualised on lateral wrist X-rays.

This normally appears to sit parallel to the anterior cortex of the radius. Anterior displacement, bowing or obliteration of this line can indicate a fracture, however, this soft-tissue sign is non-specific, and the absence of the line doesn't exclude fracture definitively. Presence of a raised fat pad in this region can also indicate; muscle strain, haematoma, inflammation, or infection (such as osteomyelitis, cellulitis or septic arthritis).

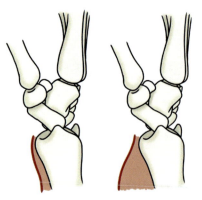

**Figure 2.31** Appearance of a normal pronator quadratus fat pad and a raised pronator quadratus fat pad.

## Ulnar variance

Refers to the relative lengths of the distal articular surfaces of the radius and ulna (independent of the length of the ulna styloid process). Lengths can be described as positive, negative or neutral. Changes to the heights of the articular surfaces can be caused by: trauma (fractures resulting in impaction/angulation or ligamentous injury), surgical intervention, growth arrest (possibly as a result of a Salter-Harris type injury) or congenital conditions (such as Madelung deformity).

Positive ulnar variance is described as the ulna sitting more than 2.5 cm beyond the distal radioulnar joint (DRUJ) This can indicate ulnar impaction syndrome, where the ulna impacts with the medial aspect of the lunate which can result in degenerative changes at both bones.

Negative ulnar variance is described as the ulna sitting more than 2.5 cm below the DRUJ. This can indicate ulnar impingement syndrome, which is where the distal ulna impinges on the medial cortex of the distal radius.

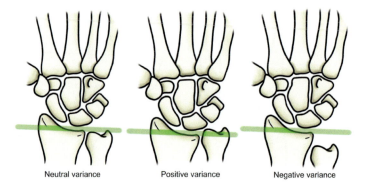

Neutral variance    Positive variance    Negative variance

**Figure 2.32** An illustration demonstrating neutral, positive, and negative ulnar variance.

# Fractures of the distal radius

Fractures of the distal radius are associated with a FOOSH particularly in older patients and are associated with high-energy mechanisms in younger patients, such as a fall from height or road traffic collisions. Patients will present with pain (resulting in reduced range of movement) along with bruising and swelling with an associated visible deformity of the wrist joint.

## Colles' fracture

The most common fracture of the distal forearm. Usually results from a FOOSH type mechanism and is commonly seen in patients over 50 years.

Classified as an extra-articular radial fracture (usually occurring 2–3 cm proximally to the articular surface) where the distal fracture fragments demonstrate dorsal (posterior) displacement/angulation. Associated avulsion fractures of the ulna styloid process are often seen.

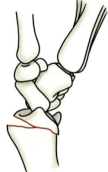

**Figure 2.33** Colles' fracture. An extra-articular fracture of the distal radius with dorsal angulation.

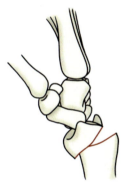

**Figure 2.34** Smith's fracture. Fracture of the distal radius with palmar angulation.

## Smith's fracture

Usually results from a fall onto the back of the hand or because of a direct blow to the hand causing forced palmar flexion.

Classified as a fracture of the distal radius with possible intra-articular extension into the radio-carpal joint. The distal fracture fragments demonstrate palmar (anterior) displacement/angulation. Sometimes referred to as a reverse Colles' fracture as the injury pattern is opposite to a Colles' fracture.

## Barton's fracture

An intra-articular fracture of the distal radius, with extension of the fracture into the radiocarpal joint (occasionally with associated dislocation). Palmar (anterior) displacement of the distal fracture fragments is more commonly seen in Barton's fractures, and if there is displacement of the distal fracture fragments there can be an associated ulna styloid avulsion fracture.

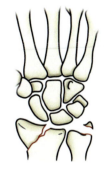

**Figure 2.35** Barton's fracture. Intra-articular fracture of the distal radius with extension towards the radio-carpal joint.

## Galeazzi fracture dislocation

A fracture of the distal third of the radius (with bony override and associated foreshortening) with an associated injury/dislocation of the distal radioulnar joint (DRUJ). However, the ulna diaphysis remains intact with no associated fracture (avulsion fracture of the ulna styloid process is possible).

Usually seen due to direct trauma to the hand or as a result of a fall onto an outstretched hand with the arm in full extension. Patients present with pain and swelling with deformity and reduced range of movement.

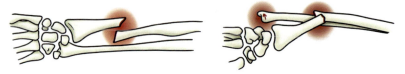

**Figure 2.36** Galeazzi fracture dislocation demonstrating a fracture of the distal radius with an associated injury at the distal radioulnar joint.

## Monteggia fracture dislocation

A fracture of the proximal third of the ulna (with bony override and associated foreshortening) with an associated dislocation of the radial head (radiocapitelar joint dislocation). More commonly seen in children (between the ages of 4–10 years) than adults.

Patients will present with pain and swelling, particularly at the elbow joint and with reduced range of movement due to the dislocation.

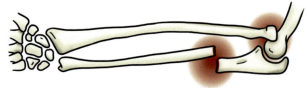

**Figure 2.37** Monteggia fracture dislocation, demonstrating a fracture of the proximal ulna with an associated dislocation of the radiocapitellar joint.

## Madelung deformity

A developmental deformity of the distal radius and carpal region caused by premature fusion of the medial aspect of the distal radial epiphysis. Premature fusion can be caused by trauma involving the growth plate (Salter-Harris fractures), infections such as osteomyelitis, vascular insufficiency or muscular disorders.

Characterised by dorsal and radial bowing of the distal radius with increased intraosseous space. The radiocarpal joint tilts towards the palmar and ulnar aspects of the distal radius with increased interosseous space, the proximal row of the carpal bones create a V shape with the lunate forced into the apex of the V. Carpal subluxation may be present with dorsal subluxation of the distal radioulnar joint (DRUJ) and positive ulnar variance.

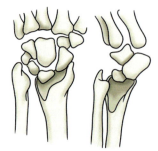

**Figure 2.38** Madelung deformity with deformity of the articular surface of the radius with displacement of the proximal carpal row.

# Systematic Assessment – Hands and Fingers

## AABCS

- Anatomy and image quality
- Alignment
- Bones
- Cartilage
- Soft tissues

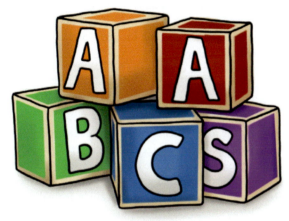

## Anatomy and image quality

Ensure the images are for the correct patient and are the most recent and up-to-date images. Is all the required anatomy

**Figure 2.39** AABCS building blocks.

demonstrated? Are the images of a good diagnostic quality? If not, consider why the images are of poor quality. This may be due to the technique used by the radiographer such as the exposures used or the patient positioning. It may be due to factors beyond the control of the radiographer such as patient body habitus or condition. External artefacts such as clothing, immobilisation aids or splints can mask anatomy or pathology.

## Alignment

Check for alignment of the **phalanges, metacarpals** and **carpal bones.** Follow a line from the distal fingertip through the phalanx, through the metacarpal and into the associated carpal bone, this line should be straight with no steps/jumps.

- 1st metacarpal articulates with the trapezium
- 2nd metacarpal articulates with the trapezoid
- 3rd metacarpal articulates with the capitate
- 4th and 5th metacarpals articulate with the hamate.

Follow the curve of the **metacarpal neck**, foreshortening or acute angulation can indicate an acute injury.

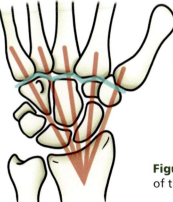

**Figure 2.40** Normal alignment of the carpometacarpal joints.

## Bones

Check each **cortex** individually – steps, breaks or acute angles in the cortical outline can indicate acute injury.

Check the **medulla** looking for areas of increased sclerosis or lucency. This may indicate a fracture or possible bone lesion.

Always assess the **edge of the film!**

## Cartilage

Check that the **joint spaces are preserved.** Degenerative changes should be noted as trauma can aggravate pain from degenerative joint changes.

Check the joint **spaces are clear** – opacity within joints may be caused by acute injury.

Assess the **articular surfaces**, which should be smooth.

Re-assess the joint **alignment**, checking for subtle subluxations.

## Soft tissues

Check for soft-tissue **swelling.**

Look for **soft-tissue damage,** e.g. splaying of the fingers can be caused by haematoma (however may also be a positional factor).

If lacerations are present, check for any evidence of **foreign body.** However, be aware that not all foreign bodies are radiopaque, e.g. not all wooden splinters will be seen on X-ray.

# Systematic Assessment – Wrist

## AABCS

- Anatomy and image quality
- Alignment
- Bones
- Cartilage
- Soft tissues

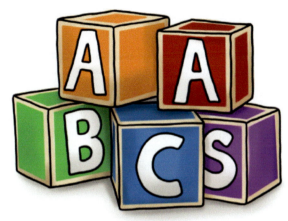

**Figure 2.41** AABCS building blocks.

## Anatomy and image quality

Ensure the images are for the correct patient and are the most recent and up-to-date images. Is all the required anatomy demonstrated? Are the images of a good diagnostic quality? If not, consider why the images are of poor quality. It may be due to the technique used by the radiographer such as the exposures used or the patient positioning. It may also be due to factors beyond the control of the radiographer such as patient body habitus or condition. External artefacts such as clothing, immobilisation aids or splints can mask anatomy or pathology.

## Alignment

Check the **carpal arcs**, each should be smooth and continuous with no steps or overlying anatomy.

Check the **lateral alignment**, especially the alignment of the radius, lunate, capitate and metacarpals.

Check the **carpal zone of vulnerability**.

Double check the **edge of film** – assessing the visualised distal radius and ulna and the proximal aspect of the metacarpals.

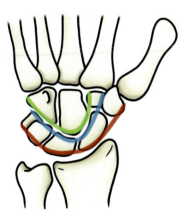

**Figure 2.42** Normal appearance and alignment of the carpal arcs.

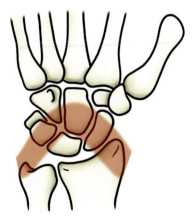

**Figure 2.43** The position of the carpal zone of vulnerability.

## Bones

Count the carpal bones; there should be 8 in an adult patient.

Check the **cortex** of each bone individually; steps, breaks or angulations of the cortex an indicate an acute fracture.

Check the **medulla** looking for areas of increased sclerosis or lucency; impacted fractures (commonly seen in FOOSH mechanism injuries) can demonstrate as a sclerotic line.

## Cartilage

Check the joint spaces are preserved and are clear.

Carpal **joint spaces** should measure approximately **2 mm** in adult patients.

Check the **Triangular Fibrocartilage complex (TFCC)** as this is a common site for avulsion type injury.

## Soft tissues

Check for soft-tissue **swelling**.

Check the **fat planes** for any sign of inflammation or swelling.

# Elbow Trauma

## Normal anatomy and alignment

The **anterior humeral line** runs along the anterior aspect of the humerus on the lateral X-ray. Normally, the line passes through the middle or the middle third of the capitellum, if this line is displaced it can indicate a supracondylar fracture.

The **radiocapitellar line** runs through the centre of the radius, extending through the joint and through the centre of the capitellum on both the AP and lateral X-ray. If the line fails to intersect the capitellum, it can indicate a radial-head dislocation.

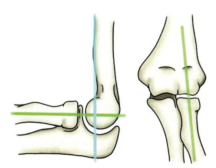

**Figure 2.44** Illustration demonstrating the normal alignment of the adult elbow – also showing the position of the anterior humeral line and the radiocapitellar line.

## Paediatric elbow

The unfused ossification centres of paediatric patients are vulnerable to particular injuries. Each ossification centre begins to develop at different ages (the trochlea and olecranon are often multicentered – don't confuse for a fracture).

Children have:

Three epiphyseal ossification centres: capitellum, trochlea and the radius

Three apophyseal ossification centres: internal and external epicondyle and the olecranon.

CRITOL – lists the most common sequence in which the ossification centres appear on X-ray:

- **Capitulum** (1 year)
- **Radial head** (3 years)
- **Internal (medial) epicondyle** (5 years)
- **Trochlea** (7 years)
- **Olecranon** (9 years)
- **Lateral epicondyle** (11 years).

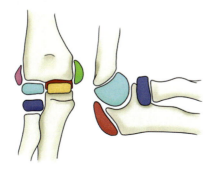

**Figure 2.45** Illustration demonstrating the normal development of the ossification centres of a paediatric elbow on X-ray imaging.

## Elbow effusion (Sail sign)

This is the elevation of the anterior and posterior fat pads to create a silhouette on a true elbow lateral X-ray. The posterior fat pad sits within the olecranon fossa and should not be visible on a normal elbow X-ray. The anterior fat pad can be seen at the anterior aspect of the distal humerus on a normal X-ray and should sit parallel to the cortex.

If there is bowing of the anterior and posterior fat pads, it indicates fluid within the joint capsule or a joint effusion. In trauma, this is caused by a haemarthrosis and indicates an intra-articular fracture even if the fracture cannot be visualised (occult fracture). Treatment and follow-up should always be considered if raised fat pads are seen. However, absence of a fat pad does not fully exclude a fracture. If the injury to the elbow joint is severe, it can rupture the joint capsule, resulting in the blood escaping the joint and preventing a haemarthrosis from developing. This prevents the fat pads from displacing and so they will not be seen on X-ray.

(a)

(b)

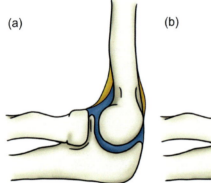
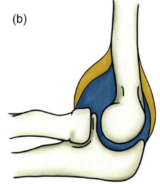

**TIP**

Posterior fat pads are not normally visible.

**Figure 2.46** (a) Shows the normal appearance of the elbow capsule and fat pads. (b) The appearance of the elbow capsule with a joint effusion present resulting in raised fat pads.

## Pulled elbow

Typically seen in young children; most commonly in patients between the ages of 1–3 years but can occur up to the age of 6 or 7 years, however this is less common. This results from pulling on the arm or hand with the elbow extended and forearm pronated, which causes the radial head to subluxate under the annular ligament. Patients present with a flexed elbow and a pronated forearm and are usually unwilling to supinate.

A pulled elbow is a clinical diagnosis where imaging may not be useful; with radiographs usually appearing normal. The radial head will easily or spontaneously relocate, and it is possible for the radiographer to 'accidently' relocate the radial head when positioning the elbow for an AP X-ray, as this involves supinating the joint.

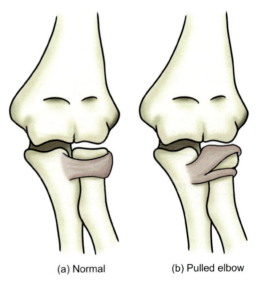

(a) Normal                    (b) Pulled elbow

**Figure 2.47** (a) Demonstrates the normal appearance of the annular ligament (b) shows the location of the annular ligament in a pulled elbow.

# Common elbow trauma

## *Supracondylar facture*

These fractures are commonly seen in paediatric patients, which can make assessment and diagnosis difficult. Supracondylar fractures can also be seen in adults, however, this is rarer. This injury typically results from a fall onto the outstretched hand (FOOSH) with hyperextension of the elbow joint. Patients present with pain, swelling and bruising (typically at the anterior aspect of the joint), with possible gross deformity. The patient will often be reluctant to move the arm, which can make assessment and imaging challenging. Neurovascular assessment should be performed to ensure there is no entrapment of nerves or blood vessels within the fracture site. If this is the case, the patient may present with loss of sensation distally with reduced range of movement, reduced distal pulse and reduced vascular perfusion.

Supracondylar fractures can be classified according to the amount of displacement of the fracture and the direction of the displacement (Gartland classification): Type I fractures demonstrate no displacement or subtle displacement. Type II fractures are displaced, however, one cortex remains intact, and Type III demonstrates full displacement.

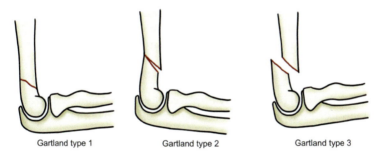

Gartland type 1        Gartland type 2        Gartland type 3

**Figure 2.48** The Gartland classifications of supracondylar fractures.

## *Lateral condyle fracture*

This is the second most commonly seen elbow fracture in paediatric patients. Injury is due to a fall onto an outstretched hand (FOOSH) causing impaction of the radial head into the lateral condyle or, as an avulsion type injury of the lateral condyle. Patients will present with pain at the lateral aspect with reduced range of movement. However, the elbow will not be as deformed as in supracondylar fracture. The bony fracture may be subtle but there will also be a cartilaginous component so the true extent of the fracture may be difficult to appreciate on X-ray. An oblique X-ray (non-routine view) may be useful for diagnosis. Accurate and timely diagnosis of lateral condyle fractures is important as they commonly displace and, without appropriate treatment (usually surgical reduction), can result in morbidity.

## *Medial epicondyle fracture*

Typically, an avulsion injury is seen in children and adolescents where patients present with pain at the medial aspect of the elbow with associated swelling and bruising. Understanding of the ossification centres and ossification sequence is important in the assessment of paediatric elbows (see CRITOL). In most patients, all ossification centres have developed by the age of 12 and missing ossification centres or ossification centres appearing in the wrong order should raise suspicion of an acute avulsion injury. Fractures of the medial epicondyle have a high association with elbow dislocations and are seen in 50% of elbow dislocations. In some cases, the medial epicondyle may avulse into the medial aspect of the elbow joint. Identification of this is important as the avulsion fragment can easily be mistaken for the trochlea ossification centre. Using CRITOL helps in these cases as the medial epicondyle ossifies before the trochlea so, if the trochlea is seen on X-ray and the medial epicondyle is not seen, an avulsion should always be considered.

## Radial head fractures

Radial head and radial neck fractures are commonly seen in all age groups; however, they are most commonly seen in patients between the ages of 20–60. These usually result from a fall onto an outstretched hand (FOOSH) with a pronated forearm. The force from the fall transmits from the wrist into the radial head. Patients will present with swelling and pain, particularly at the lateral aspect of the elbow joint, with reduced range of movement affecting pronation and supination.

In children, the fracture tends to involve the radial neck and is commonly known as a Salter-Harris type II fracture. Radial head and neck fractures can be very subtle and a thorough assessment of the lateral X-ray for a joint effusion (sail sign) is vital as this can indicate the presence of a subtle or an occult fracture and should be treated appropriately if there is clinical suspicion.

Radial head fractures can be classified using the Mason classification system:

- **Type I:** non-displaced or minimally displaced (less than 2 mm) fracture
- **Type II:** displaced fracture fragment (greater than 2 mm) with possible angulation
- **Type III:** comminuted fracture with displacement
- **Type IV:** radial head fracture with an associated dislocation.

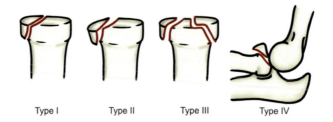

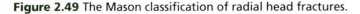
Type I     Type II     Type III     Type IV

**Figure 2.49** The Mason classification of radial head fractures.

## Olecranon fracture

This fracture is seen as the result of low-energy trauma in the elderly and high-energy trauma in younger patients. It is usually obvious both clinically and radiologically and can result from a fall onto an outstretched hand/arm with the elbow in flexion, direct blow or avulsion injury and is usually as a result of triceps contraction. Patients present with swelling at the posterior aspect of the elbow joint, pain, reduced range of movement with an inability to extend the arm and a palpable fracture fragment. Treatment usually involves open reduction and internal fixation (ORIF).

## Elbow dislocations

The elbow joint is the second most commonly dislocated joint in adults (most common in children) and are typically seen as a result of a FOOSH with the arm in extension. Patients will present with pain, swelling and deformity at the elbow joint.

Dislocations of the elbow joint can be described according to the movement of the ulna in relation to the distal humerus, these include: posterior dislocation, anterior dislocation, radial/lateral dislocation, ulna/medical dislocation or divergent dislocations.

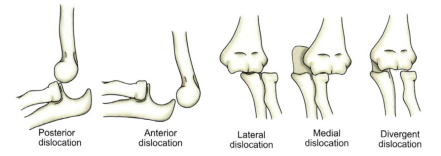

| Posterior dislocation | Anterior dislocation | Lateral dislocation | Medial dislocation | Divergent dislocation |

**Figure 2.50** Different types of elbow dislocations.

These dislocations can be further classified as simple or complex. Simple dislocations involve the dislocation of an elbow joint with no associated fractures and are the most common type of elbow dislocation. Complex dislocations also involve associated fractures and tend to demonstrate instability.

The terrible triad of injuries of the elbow (Figure 2.51) is an example of a complex elbow dislocation. These injuries are typically seen in adult patients and involve a dislocation of the elbow joint with associated fractures of the coronoid process and the radial head or neck. The dislocation is often a posterior dislocation with associated injury of the lateral collateral ligament.

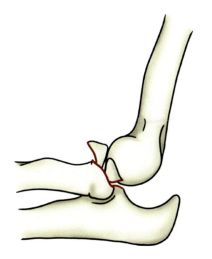

**Figure 2.51** The pattern of a 'terrible triad' injury involving a dislocation of the elbow joint with associated coronoid process and radial head/neck fractures.

## Systematic Assessment of the Elbow

### AABCS

- Anatomy and image quality
- Alignment
- Bones
- Cartilage
- Soft tissues

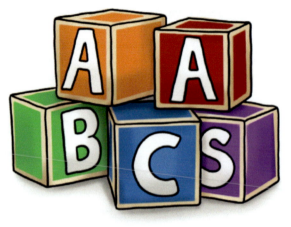

### Anatomy and image quality

Ensure the images are for the correct patient and are the most recent and up-to-date. Is all the required anatomy demonstrated?

**Figure 2.52** AABCS building blocks.

Are the images of a good diagnostic quality? If they are not, consider why the images are of poor quality. It may be due to the technique used by the radiographer such as exposures used or patient positioning. It could also be due to factors beyond the control of the radiographer such as patient body habitus or condition. External artefacts such as clothing or immobilisation aids can also mask anatomy or pathology.

### Alignment

Check the **alignment**, checking the anterior humeral line. Ensure this line runs through the middle or the middle third of the capitellum, then check the radiocapitellar line making sure it runs through the centre of the radius, through the joint and through the centre of the capitellum on both the AP and lateral X-ray.

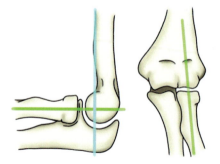

**Figure 2.53** Illustration demonstrating the normal alignment of the adult elbow – also showing the position of the anterior humeral line and the radiocapitellar line.

### Bones

Check the **cortex** of each bone individually; steps, breaks or angulations of the cortex an indicate an acute fracture.

Check the **medulla** looking for areas of increased sclerosis or lucency.

In paediatric patients, ensure the development of the unfused apophysis are in keeping with the age of the patient using **CRITOL – 1 Capitulum** (1 year), **2 Radial head** (3 years), **3 Internal (medial) epicondyle** (5 years), **4 Trochlea** (7 years), **5 Olecranon** (9 years), **6 Lateral epicondyle** (11 years).

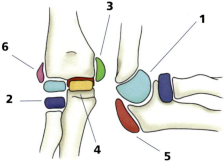

**Figure 2.54** Illustration demonstrating the normal development of the ossification centres of a paediatric elbow on X-ray imaging.

## Cartilage

Check the joint spaces are preserved and are clear.

## Soft tissues

Check for soft-tissue **swelling.**

Check the **anterior and posterior fat pads.** On normal X-ray, the anterior fat pad should be visible but will sit parallel to the anterior cortex of the humerus; the posterior fat pad should not be seen. If the anterior fat pad is raised with a raised posterior fat pad, consider a fracture even if one cannot be seen, and treat accordingly.

(a)        (b)

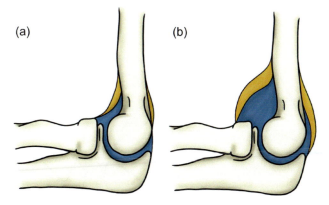

**Figure 2.55** (a) Shows the normal appearance of the elbow capsule and fat pads. (b) The appearance of the elbow capsule with a joint effusion present resulting in raised fat pads.

## Shoulder Girdle

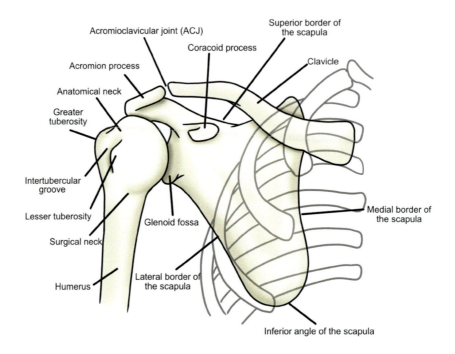

Figure 2.56 Anatomy of the shoulder – anterior aspect.

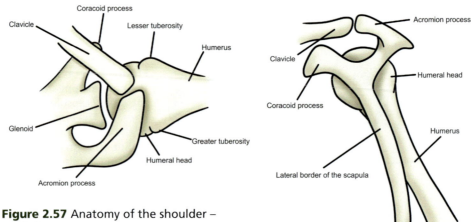

**Figure 2.57** Anatomy of the shoulder – axial view.

**Figure 2.58** Anatomy of the shoulder – Y-view.

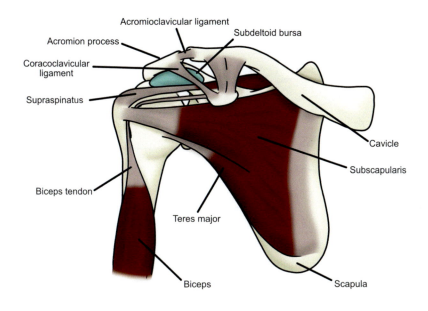

**Figure 2.59** Anatomy of the shoulder muscles – anterior aspect.

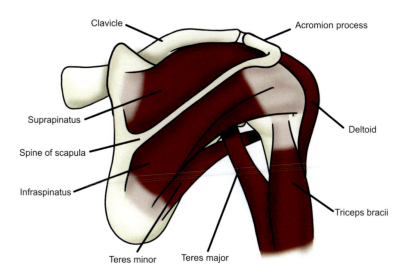

**Figure 2.60** Anatomy of the shoulder muscles – posterior aspect.

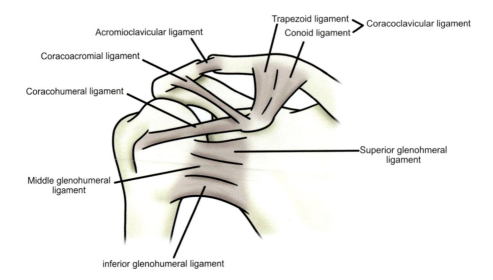

Figure 2.61 Anatomy of the shoulder ligaments and tendons.

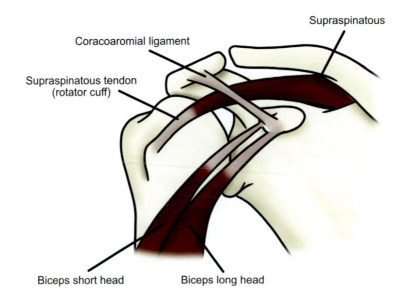

Figure 2.62 Anatomy of the shoulder ligaments and tendons.

# Shoulder Trauma

The shoulder is the most mobile joint in the body. In addition to this, the glenoid cavity is relatively shallow, which results in the shoulder joint being the most common joint to subluxate/dislocate (approximately 50% of all dislocations occur at the shoulder).

> **TIP**
>
> As the shoulder is the most mobile joint, it is also the easiest to dislocate.

## Shoulder alignment and measurements

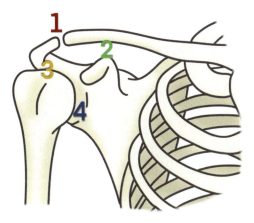

**Figure 2.63** Illustration showing the normal alignment and measurements of the shoulder –
1 = Acromioclavicular joint,
2 = Coracoclavicular ligament,
3 = Subacromial space,
4 = Glenohumeral joint.

### 1. Acromioclavicular joint

The inferior aspect of the acromion should align with the inferior aspect of the lateral end of the clavicle. If the alignment is lost, consider subluxation/dislocation of the acromioclavicular joint (ACJ) with associated ligamentous injury. A normal ACJ distance should measure 5–8 mm. However, it can be narrower in the elderly.

### 2. Coracoclavicular joint

This can be used alongside the ACJ alignment to assess for ligamentous injury. The normal distance of the coracoclavicular joint should be between 10–13 mm, with increased distance indicating ligamentous injury.

### 3. Subacromial space

A measurement taken from the inferior aspect of the acromion process to the superior aspect of the humeral head. Normal measurement range is 8–12 mm. If the distance is increased, it is indicative of a shoulder subluxation/dislocation. However, this can also be caused by an effusion or haemarthrosis within the joint (pseudo-subluxation). If the distance is reduced, this can indicate rotator cuff arthropathy.

### 4. Glenohumeral joint

The humerus should lie within the glenoid fossa. The distance between the humeral head and the glenoid rim should be equal and loss of alignment or overlap can indicate joint dislocation.

## Shoulder dislocations

### Anterior shoulder dislocation

The anterior is the most common form of shoulder dislocation, accounting for approximately 95%. It usually results from forced abduction, external rotation and extension. Patients will present with pain, reduced range of movement/sensation and deformity of the affected shoulder. The shoulder will lose its normal rounded appearance and will appear squared with external rotation and abduction, with the humeral head palpable anteriorly. This can also cause injury to the axillary nerve, so function should also be assessed clinically. On X-ray, the humeral head will appear to overlap with the glenoid; with the humeral head most commonly seen sitting in a sub-coracoid position. However, sub-glenoid, sub-clavicular and intrathoracic (very rare) positions can also be seen.

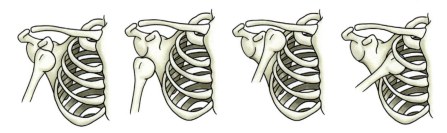

**Figure 2.64** Four types of anterior shoulder dislocation – sub-coracoid position, sub-glenoid, sub-clavicular and intrathoracic.

> **TIP**
>
> Axillary nerve injuries are associated with shoulder dislocations. Remember to assess its distribution, the 'regimental badge' area.

### Posterior shoulder dislocation

This is not as common as anterior dislocations (2–4%). It usually results from internal rotation with the arm in abduction, forcing the humeral head posteriorly and is commonly seen following a seizure. Posterior dislocations may not be as clinically obvious as anterior dislocations, but the patient will present with pain, reduced range of movement with the arm in fixed adduction and internal rotation. The shoulder will lose its normal rounded appearance with prominence at the posterior aspect and possible posteriorly palpable humeral head.

Posterior dislocations can be subtle on AP X-ray. However, the AP view can demonstrate the following features:

- **Lightbulb sign:** internal rotation of the humeral head makes it appear more rounded.
- **Trough line sign:** dense vertical line in the medial humeral head due to the humeral head impacting.

The axial view is considered the gold standard for detection of posterior shoulder dislocations with the humeral head sitting in an obvious posterior position.

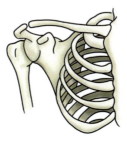

**Figure 2.65** A posterior shoulder dislocation.

## *Inferior shoulder dislocation*

Also known as Luxatio Erecta, this is the least common form of shoulder dislocation, accounting for less than 1% of the total. It is typically associated with high-energy trauma resulting in forced hyper-extension. Patients present with pain, reduced range of movement and deformity of the shoulder, with the arm in fixed abduction, held upwards, in a saluting position.

There is a high association with further injury following an inferior shoulder dislocation, including soft-tissue injury, ligamentous and tendon damage (possible capsule rupture) and neurovascular injury. A thorough neurovascular assessment is required pre- and post-reduction to assess for associated injury.

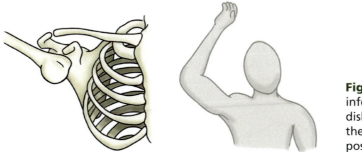

**Figure 2.66** An inferior shoulder dislocation with the typical saluting position.

## Bankart lesion

A Bankart lesion is an injury to the anteroinferior aspect of the glenoid labrum and is an associated complication of anterior shoulder dislocations. Bankart lesions occur as the humeral head impacts on the anteroinferior aspect of the glenoid labrum during an anterior dislocation resulting in injury to this region of the glenoid labrum or glenoid rim. Soft-tissue injury only involving the glenoid labrum is more common than a 'bony Bankart' lesion which involves an associated fracture fragment at the anteroinferior aspect of the glenoid rim.

On X-ray, a bony Bankart lesion will appear as a curvilinear or triangular-shaped fracture fragment at the anteroinferior aspect of the glenoid rim. Bankart lesions, without an associated fracture, may be occult and MRI can be used to fully appreciate the soft-tissue damage that has occurred.

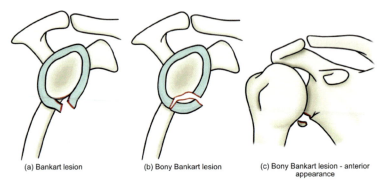

(a) Bankart lesion    (b) Bony Bankart lesion    (c) Bony Bankart lesion - anterior appearance

**Figure 2.67** Illustration showing the appearance of (a) Bankart lesion, (b) bony Bankart lesion and (c) the anterior appearance of a bony Bankart lesion.

**TIP**

MRI may be needed to fully appreciate the extent of this injury.

## Hill-Sachs deformity

A Hill-Sachs deformity is a depression-type fracture at the posterolateral aspect of the humeral head caused by anterior shoulder dislocation, with repeated dislocations resulting in a larger Hill-Sachs deformity. As the humeral head dislocates anteriorly, the humeral head impacts with the anterior aspect of the glenoid causing a bony defect at the posterolateral aspect of the humeral head. In patients where there is a Hill-Sachs deformity, there is an association with Bankart lesions. If a Hill-Sachs is identified, it is important to thoroughly assess the anteroinferior aspect of the glenoid for an associated Bankart lesion.

On X-ray, a Hill-Sachs deformity will present as a concave depression at the posterolateral aspect of the humeral head, which can be seen best on the AP view.

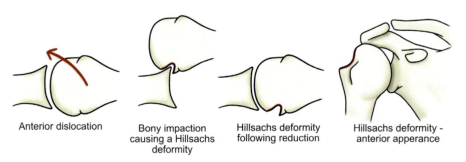

Anterior dislocation    Bony impaction causing a Hillsachs deformity    Hillsachs deformity following reduction    Hillsachs deformity - anterior apperance

**Figure 2.68** The process of the formation of a Hill-Sachs deformity – anterior dislocation with impaction of the humeral head on the glenoid.

## Acromioclavicular joint injury

This is a commonly seen ligamentous injury which typically occurs following trauma such as a fall onto the apex of the shoulder, a FOOSH or because of a direct blow to the shoulder and is commonly seen as a result of contact sport injury. Patients present with pain, particularly over the AC joint, and localised swelling and deformity may also be present.

X-rays are used to assess the acromioclavicular and coracoclavicular ligaments. In a normal ACJ, the joint should measure between 5–8 mm (it may be narrower in elderly patients) and the inferior aspect of the acromion should align with the inferior aspect of the lateral end of the clavicle. If there is disruption to either of these areas, a ligamentous injury should be considered.

## Classification of acromioclavicular joint injury (Rockwood classification)

The Rockwood classification takes into account the acromioclavicular and coracoclavicular ligaments, whilst considering the direction of the dislocation.

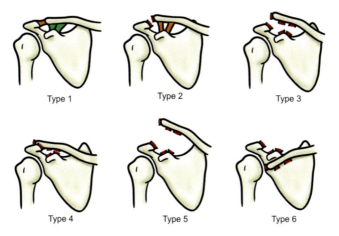

Type 1        Type 2        Type 3

Type 4        Type 5        Type 6

**Figure 2.69** The Rockwood classification of acromioclavicular joint injury.

A breakdown of the Rockwood classification is as follows:

- **Type 1**: Acromioclavicular ligament (ACL) mild sprain, the coracoclavicular ligament (CCL) and joint capsule remains intact. No associated muscle damage.
- **Type 2**: Clavicle slightly raised. ACL ruptured, CCL sprained, and the joint capsule is ruptured. The deltoid and trapezius muscles are minimally detached.
- **Type 3**: Clavicle superiorly raised, coracoclavicular distance is increased (but measures less than twice normal distance). The ACL, CCL and joint capsules are ruptured. The deltoid and trapezius muscles are detached.
- **Type 4**: Clavicle displaced posteriorly onto the trapezoid. ACL, CCL and joint capsule ruptured. The deltoid and trapezius muscles are detached.

- **Type 5**: Clavicle significantly raised with the coracoclavicular distance more than double normal distance. ACL, CCL and joint capsule ruptured. The deltoid and trapezius muscles are detached.
- **Type 6**: Clavicle inferiorly displaced behind the coracobrachialis and biceps tendon = RARE. ACL, CCL and joint capsule ruptured. The deltoid and trapezius muscles are detached.

## Clavicle fractures

Fractures of the clavicle are relatively common, accounting for approximately 2–4% of all adult fractures. The midshaft of the clavicle is the most common location to see a fracture and is usually the result of a direct blow such as that following a fall onto the lateral aspect of the shoulder or as a result of contact sports. Fractures of the lateral aspect of the clavicle are more commonly seen in the elderly, osteoporotic patient and are also a result of a direct blow to this region. In an elderly patient, they are commonly associated with falls. Fractures of the medial aspect of the clavicle are rare and can be difficult to visualise on X-ray due to overlying rib anatomy so, if a medial clavicle fracture is clinically suspected, thorough inspection of this region on X-ray is crucial.

Patients will present with anterior shoulder pain with point tenderness at the fracture site. Bruising and swelling may be present and in displaced fractures skin tenting may be present.

## Classification of clavicle fractures (Neer classification)

The Neer classification looks at the stability of the fracture with consideration for associated ligamentous injury:

- **Type 1**: fracture site is at the lateral aspect of the coracoclavicular ligament with minimal displacement. Conoid and trapezoid ligaments remain intact.
- **Type 2a**: fracture is medial to the coracoclavicular ligament, with minimal displacement of the fracture site. Conoid and trapezoid ligaments are intact. Considered an unstable injury with a 56% non union rate if treated non-operatively.
- **Type 2b**: Two fracture patterns. The fracture site is between the coracoclavicular ligament with the conoid ligament ruptured, however the trapezoid ligament remains intact. Or the fracture is lateral to the coracoclavicular ligament with both the conoid and trapezoid ligaments ruptured. Medial clavicle displacement. Considered an unstable fracture with a non union rate of 30–45% with non-operative treatment.
- **Type 3**: An intra-articular fracture extending into the acromioclavicular joint with minimal displacement. Conoid and trapezoid ligaments remain intact. Considered a stable injury, however secondary (post-traumatic) osteoarthritis may develop.
- **Type 4**: Occurs in the immature skeleton. Physeal fracture with lateral clavicle displacement (occurs through a superior tear in the periosteum). Conoid and trapezoid ligaments remain intact. Considered a stable injury.
- **Type 5**: Comminuted fracture with significant medial displacement Conoid and trapezoid ligaments remain intact. Considered an unstable injury.

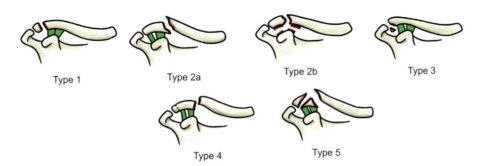
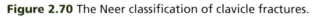

**Figure 2.70** The Neer classification of clavicle fractures.

## Proximal humerus fractures

Proximal humerus fractures are common fracture, typically seen in osteoporotic or elderly patients. They are usually the result of a low-energy mechanism such as a FOOSH or a direct fall onto the shoulder. In younger patients, proximal humerus fractures are associated with higher energy mechanisms of injury such as road traffic collisions or falls from height. Patients present with reduced range of movement, pain and swelling with bruising over the anterior aspect of the chest and arm.

## Classification of proximal humerus fractures (Neer classification)

### One-part fractures

These can involve multiple fracture lines. However, there is no or very little displacement, and they account for approximately 70–80% of all proximal humeral fractures. These are usually treated conservatively.

### Two-part fractures

These can involve multiple fracture lines, with slight displacement of one fracture fragment. There are four types: surgical neck fracture, greater tuberosity fractures (frequently seen with anterior displacement), anatomical neck fractures and lesser tuberosity fractures (uncommon). These account for approximately 20% of all proximal humerus fractures.

### Three-part fractures

These fractures involve multiple parts with displacement of two fracture fragments. The most common three-part fractures involve the diaphysis and greater tuberosity with displacement in relation to the lesser tuberosity and articular surface. Three-part fractures account for approximately 5% of proximal humerus fractures.

### Four-part fractures

These form an uncommon fracture pattern, accounting for less than 1% of proximal humerus fractures. Four-part fractures are usually displaced with poor non-operative results and a high incidence of osteonecrosis.

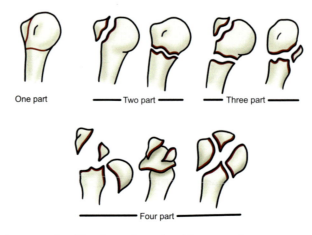

**Figure 2.71** The Neer classification of proximal humerus fractures.

# Systematic Assessment – Shoulder

## AABCS

- Anatomy and image quality
- Alignment
- Bones
- Cartilage
- Soft tissues

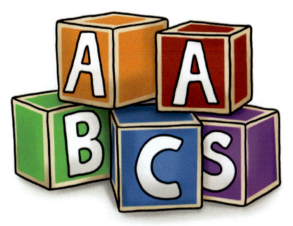

**Figure 2.72** AABCS building blocks.

## Anatomy and image quality

Ensure the images are for the correct patient and are the most recent and up-to-date images. Is all the required anatomy demonstrated? Are the images of a good diagnostic quality? If they are not, consider why – it may be due to the technique used by the radiographer such as exposures used or patient positioning. It may also be due to factors beyond the control of the radiographer such as patient body habitus or condition. External artefacts such as clothing, immobilisation aids or splints can mask anatomy or pathology.

## Alignment

Check all the joints:

**Glenohumeral joint:** articular surface should be in contact with the glenoid.

**Acromioclavicular joint:** assess the ligament – **5–8 mm** is a normal measurement. It should be aligned at the **inferior aspect**. Be aware of possible traumatic or arthritic bony lysis.

**Coracoclavicular ligament: 10–13 mm** is considered a normal measurement.

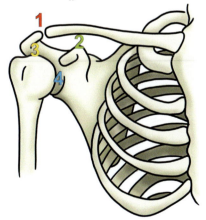

**Figure 2.73** Illustration showing the normal alignment and measurements of the shoulder – 1 = Acromioclavicular joint, 2 = Coracoclavicular ligament, 3 = Subacromial space, 4 = Glenohumeral joint.

## Bones and cartilage

It is important to assess the bones and the cartilage together due to anatomy.

Assess the shape of the **humeral head.** Imaging should be performed with the hand in external rotation to put the humeral head into profile. This should have a slight curve at the neck (this is a point of weakness due to anisotropic bony properties). Check for the lightbulb sign – consider if it is a positional appearance or due to a posterior dislocation.

Check the **medulla** assessing for increased sclerosis or lucency.

Be aware of **physeal plate lines** and **ossification centres** in paediatric patients. The physeal line is located at the base of the humeral head near the neck curvature and can mimic a fracture. The humeral head has two ossification centres (the humeral head and greater tuberosity). Ossification of the coracoid and acromion should be thin and uniform.

**Scapula:** assessment can be difficult due to overlying anatomy. However, make sure you can fully visualise all cortexes.

**Clavicle:** most commonly fractured bone in paediatrics. The curved shape causes the bone to be weak. Midshaft fractures are the most common, medial fractures are rare and can be difficult to diagnose due to overlying anatomy.

## Soft tissues

Check for lucency in the shoulder capsule as this may represent a **lipohaemarthrosis** which can indicate a fracture. However, the presence of a subtle curvilinear lucency at the cortex of the humeral head is normal.

**Rotator cuff calcifications:** all tendons in and around the humeral head are active, stress on these structures can cause calcifications to develop and are commonly seen in supraspinatus tendon calcification (**calcific tendinopathy**).

**TIP**

When assessing shoulder and clavicle X-rays, don't forget to assess the whole image. Rib fractures and pneumothoraces can be easily missed.

# Chapter 3

# Lower Limb

## Overview

This chapter will cover a review of the lower limb, including the femur, tibia and fibula, and foot along with an assessment of the knee and ankle joints. This chapter begins with an overview of the bony anatomy of the lower limb, while also introducing some soft-tissue anatomy of muscles and ligaments. Following this, we will cover common mechanisms of injury, with associated fracture patterns and classifications of injury types. Chronic conditions, such as degenerative change, will be introduced followed by a systematic review technique for each region.

## Anatomy

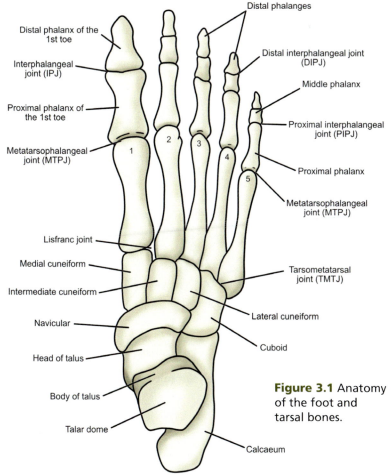

**Figure 3.1** Anatomy of the foot and tarsal bones.

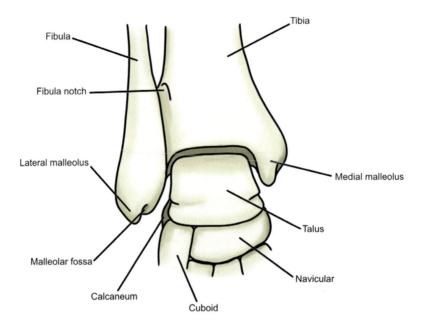

**Figure 3.2** Anatomy of the ankle joint (anterior aspect).

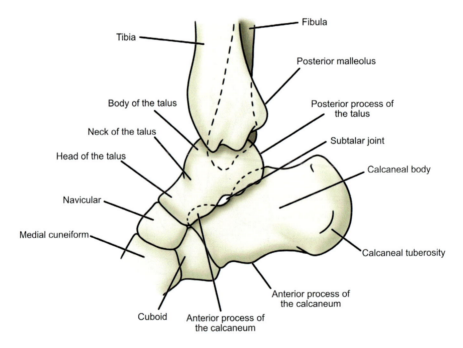

**Figure 3.3** Anatomy of the ankle joint (medial aspect).

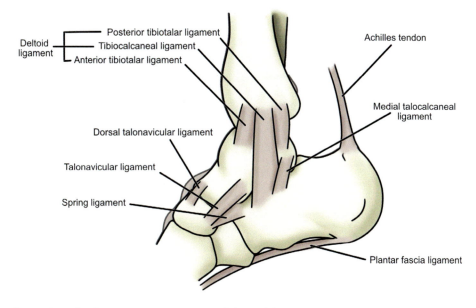

Deltoid ligament:
- Posterior tibiotalar ligament
- Tibiocalcaneal ligament
- Anterior tibiotalar ligament

Achilles tendon

Medial talocalcaneal ligament

Dorsal talonavicular ligament

Talonavicular ligament

Spring ligament

Plantar fascia ligament

**Figure 3.4** The ligamentous anatomy of the ankle joint (medial aspect).

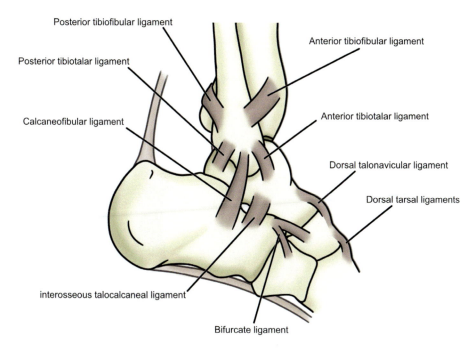

Posterior tibiofibular ligament

Anterior tibiofibular ligament

Posterior tibiotalar ligament

Calcaneofibular ligament

Anterior tibiotalar ligament

Dorsal talonavicular ligament

Dorsal tarsal ligaments

interosseous talocalcaneal ligament

Bifurcate ligament

**Figure 3.5** The ligamentous anatomy of the ankle joint (lateral aspect).

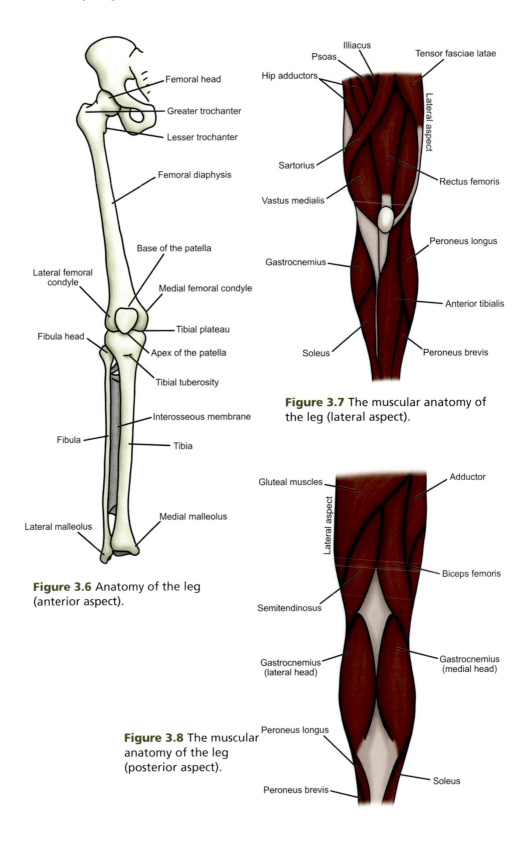

Femoral head

Greater trochanter

Lesser trochanter

Femoral diaphysis

Base of the patella

Lateral femoral condyle

Medial femoral condyle

Tibial plateau

Fibula head

Apex of the patella

Tibial tuberosity

Interosseous membrane

Fibula

Tibia

Lateral malleolus

Medial malleolus

**Figure 3.6** Anatomy of the leg (anterior aspect).

Illiacus

Psoas

Hip adductors

Tensor fasciae latae

Lateral aspect

Sartorius

Rectus femoris

Vastus medialis

Peroneus longus

Gastrocnemius

Anterior tibialis

Soleus

Peroneus brevis

**Figure 3.7** The muscular anatomy of the leg (lateral aspect).

Gluteal muscles

Adductor

Lateral aspect

Biceps femoris

Semitendinosus

Gastrocnemius (lateral head)

Gastrocnemius (medial head)

Peroneus longus

Soleus

**Figure 3.8** The muscular anatomy of the leg (posterior aspect).

Peroneus brevis

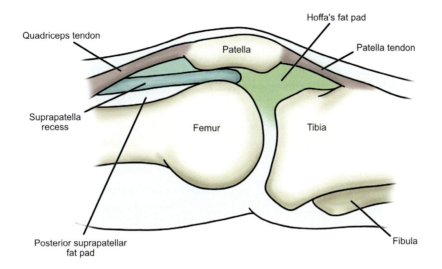

Hoffa's fat pad

Quadriceps tendon

Patella

Patella tendon

Suprapatella
recess

Femur

Tibia

Posterior suprapatellar
fat pad

Fibula

**Figure 3.9** Anatomy of the knee joint (lateral aspect).

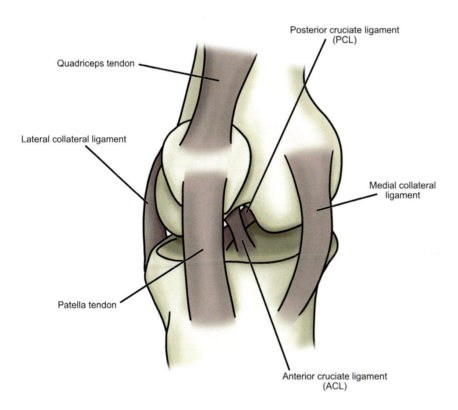

Posterior cruciate ligament
(PCL)

Quadriceps tendon

Lateral collateral ligament

Medial collateral
ligament

Patella tendon

Anterior cruciate ligament
(ACL)

**Figure 3.10** The ligamentous anatomy of the knee joint.

# Knee Trauma

## Ottawa knee rules

This is a clinical decision tool to help determine the need for diagnostic imaging. Patients who present with any of the following criteria require imaging according to the Ottawa rules:

- Patients over the age of 55 presenting with trauma to the knee.
- Isolated tenderness to the patella.
- Tenderness to the fibula head.
- Inability to flex to 90°.
- Inability to weight bear (immediately after trauma or on admission to A&E).

## Knee soft tissues

Normally, the suprapatellar fat pad is divided in two by a soft-tissue density (suprapatellar recess). This should normally measure 5 mm or less. If there is some form of soft-tissue injury (meniscal/ligamentous), this may extend to form a joint effusion. The majority of knee injuries affect the soft tissues with no bony injury.

When there is an intra-articular fracture involving the knee, blood and bone marrow (containing fat) leak into the joint. This causes a fat/blood fluid level to form, called a lipohaemarthrosis. The fat will sit on top of the dense blood, creating a horizontal line on a supine knee X-ray (all trauma knee X-rays should be performed supine, using a horizontal beam technique to allow a lipohaemarthrosis to form). The presence of lipohaemarthrosis Indicates a fracture, even if it can't be visualised on X-ray (occult fracture).

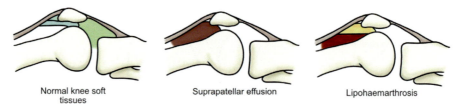

Normal knee soft tissues     Suprapatellar effusion     Lipohaemarthrosis

**Figure 3.11** The appearance of normal knee soft tissues, a suprapatellar effusion and a lipohaemarthrosis.

> ## TIP
> Presence of a lipohaemarthrosis indicates a fracture even if one is not visualised.

## Patella injury

Fractures of the patella often occur from a direct impact to the knee such as a fall onto a flexed knee or following a road traffic collision with the knee hitting the dashboard. Patella fractures can also be due to tension mechanisms caused by sudden contraction of the quadriceps. Patients will present with pain, swelling, reduced range of movement, laceration, haemarthrosis and a palpable fracture site.

Fractures of the patella tend to be vertical or transverse involving the body of the patella. Skyline X-ray views are contraindicated when the fractures have a transverse orientation. When the knee is bent to perform this view, the fracture is at risk of displacing due to the position of the patella and the quadriceps tendon insertion points.

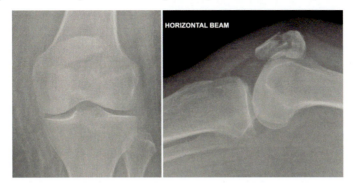

**Figure 3.12** X-ray demonstrating a transverse fracture of the patella. © 2022 University Hospitals of North Midlands NHS Trust. All rights reserved.

> ## TIP
> Skyline views are contraindicated in patella fractures due to the risk of worsening the injury.

## Bipartite patella

Bipartite patellae are normal variants caused by secondary ossification centres. The ossification centres tend to occur in characteristic locations, usually within the superolateral aspect of the patella. It will appear as a well corticated bony density. Some bipartite patellas may have a multi-fragmented appearance and are known as multipartite patella.

These normal variants are often found incidentally and may present asymptomatically. However, some patients may present with anterior knee pain following trauma to the knee or overuse which makes diagnosis difficult.

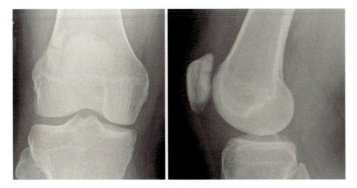

**Figure 3.13** X-ray demonstrating a multipartite patella – an asymptomatic normal variant. © 2022 University Hospitals of North Midlands NHS Trust. All rights reserved.

## Insall-Salvati ratio

This is the ratio between the length of the patella tendon and the length of the patella. The measurement should be taken with the knee flexed at 30°. The patella tendon length is divided by the patella length to give the Insall-Salvati ratio. For example, if the patella tendon = 3.97 cm and the patella measures 4.58 cm; 3.97 ÷ 4.58 = 0.8668.

The normal ratio should be between 0.8–1.2. If the ratio is less than 0.8, the patella is low lying = patella baja, if the ratio is greater than 1.2, the patella is high riding = patella alta.

> **TIP**
>
> Patella **Alta** = **Above**
> Patella **Baja** = **Below**

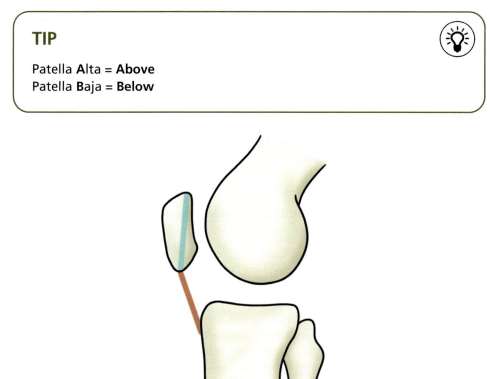

**Figure 3.14** Illustration demonstrating the alignment of the patella, with the patella length demonstrated in blue and the patella tendon length demonstrated in red.

Patella baja and alta can both present with anterior knee pain and can indicate several pathologies. Patella alta can indicate a rupture of the patella tendon or dislocation but can also be associated with chronic conditions such as Osgood-Schlatter's disease, Sinding-Larsen-Johansson disease or congenital defects. Patella baja can indicate rupture of the quadriceps or dislocation and can be seen following a total knee replacement or ACL repair due to shortening of the patella tendon. Patella baja is also commonly seen in congenital conditions such as achondroplasia.

# Knee avulsion fractures

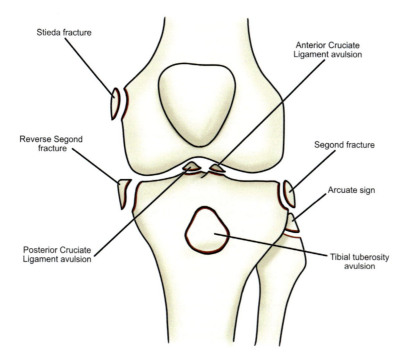

**Figure 3.15** An illustration of commonly seen avulsion fractures of the knee; Stieda fracture, reverse segond fracture, segond fracture, posterior cruciate ligament avulsion, anterior cruciate ligament avulsion, arcuate sign and tibial tuberosity avulsion.

## Stieda fracture

This results from stress away from the midline with valgus instability. Fracture fragment is seen at the medial femoral condyle, with avulsion of the attachment point of the medial collateral ligaments (MCL). It is associated with ACL rupture with possible medial tibiofemoral joint space widening on X-ray.

## Reverse segond fracture

This results from external rotation with stress away from the midline and is associated with high-energy mechanisms. A linear fracture fragment can be seen at the medial aspect of the tibial plateau, which is associated with an avulsion of the MCL.

## Posterior cruciate ligament (PCL) avulsion

This results from posterior force against the tibia with a flexed knee. It is commonly seen in motorbike accidents and road traffic collisions (RTCs) but can also be seen following a sport injury involving hyperflexion of the knee joint on a plantarflexed foot. PCL avulsion is more commonly seen at the tibial aspect and usually involves a fracture of the posterior tibial eminence or tibial articular surface (which will be best visualised on the lateral projection).

### *Anterior cruciate ligament (ACL) avulsion*

This results from knee joint hyper-extension or following a direct blow to a knee in flexion. ACL avulsion is more commonly seen at the tibial aspect and usually involves a fracture of the tibial eminence. Due to the disruption of the ACL, the tibia may demonstrate slight anterior displacement in relation to the femur on the lateral view, indicating joint instability.

### *Segond fracture*

This results from internal rotation with stress towards the midline and can be caused by a fall, a direct blow or following a sporting injury (most commonly seen in football, basketball and skiing). A linear or curvilinear fracture fragment is seen at the lateral aspect of the tibial plateau. The avulsion fragment is associated with the lateral collateral ligament and, although the fracture fragment may appear small on X-ray, it is linked with extensive ligamentous injury. Associated injury to the ACL is commonly seen with segond fractures.

### *Arcuate sign*

This results from a direct blow to the anterior/medial aspect of an extended or hyper-extended knee, with internal rotation or from a high-mechanism injury involving a knee joint dislocation. It usually results in a small, horizontally orientated fracture of the fibula head at the insertion point of the arcuate ligament complex. Injury to this region can result in knee joint instability.

### *Tibial tuberosity avulsion*

This results from forced flexion of the knee or from significant contraction of the quadriceps. It is typically seen when landing from a jump and is most frequently seen in the immature skeleton. X-rays will demonstrate a fracture involving the anterior aspect of the tibial tuberosity with widening of the apophysis and patella alta.

## Knee soft-tissue injury

Soft-tissue injury to the knee is common in the acute setting and is typically seen after sporting injuries (such as football or rugby). It is caused by:

- Hyperflexion, hyper-extension, direct blow, or a fall can result in damage to the cruciate ligaments
- Varus and valgus forces can result in collateral ligament injury
- A twisting-type mechanism can cause injury to the meniscus
- Sudden muscular contraction can result in muscular rupture, most commonly involving the quadriceps.

## Pellegrini-Stieda lesion

This is a post-traumatic chronic classification within the MCL which can indicate previous injury to the MCL. This characteristically appears on X-ray as a linear or curvilinear calcification parallel to the medial condyle. The majority of patients will present asymptomatically with the lesion being found incidentally. However, occasionally the patient will experience medial knee pain known as Pellegrini-Stieda syndrome.

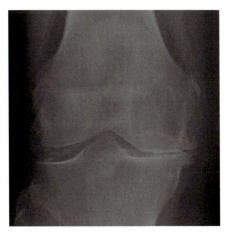

**Figure 3.16** X-ray demonstrating a Pellegrini-Stieda lesion – a chronic calcification within the medial collateral ligament. © 2022 University Hospitals of North Midlands NHS Trust. All rights reserved.

## Osteochondral injury

Osteochondral fractures involve injury to the articular surface and subchondral bone and can be seen in the femoral condyles, tibial plateau and patella. These fractures are usually occult on plain film X-ray due to the involvement of the cartilaginous element of the joint and may require MR imaging for diagnosis. However, if the fracture fragment has become displaced, plain film imaging may be able to detect the fracture. X-rays will show a fracture line with extension towards the articular surface, subchondral bone depression and irregularity of the articular surface.

Osteochondritis dissecans (OCD) is a condition affecting the joints and is most commonly seen in the knee but can also affect other joints such as the ankle and elbow. It is most commonly seen in adolescents and young adults. Reduced blood supply to the bone resulting in localised avascular necrosis (AVN) causes a bone fragment (usually ovoid in shape) to become detached from the healthy bone/cartilage forming an OCD lesion. The exact cause of OCD is unknown, however, repetitive microtrauma and genetic predisposition may have an impact. The lesion appears as a subarticular lucency with sclerotic margins. Within the lucency sits an ovoid bone segment (an area of AVN) and this is characteristically seen within the lateral femoral condyle (also seen in the capitellum and talus).

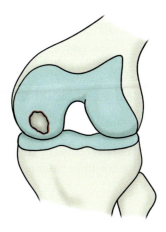

**Figure 3.17** Osteochondral injury

### Tibial plateau fractures

These are associated with high-energy mechanisms such as such as a fall from height which is more frequently seen in younger patients. In older patients with a history of osteoporosis depression-type fractures are more commonly seen.

Fractures of the lateral tibial plateau are most commonly seen in lower force mechanisms and are associated with valgus forces in high-energy mechanisms. Varus forces are associated with medial tibial plateau fractures and axial loading (commonly seen in falls from height) and can result in bicondylar fractures. Fractures of the tibial plateau are often associated with soft-tissue injury, such as meniscal or ligamentous injury, and fractures involving the lateral or medial aspect of the tibial plateau may present with injury to the opposite ligaments.

Patients will present with pain and tenderness, swelling, haemarthrosis, reduced range of movement with an inability to weight bear and ligamentous instability.

When assessing the tibial plateau on X-ray, be aware that the articular surface is angled approximately 10° to 15° posteroinferiorly, which may result in occult fractures of the tibial plateau (however, a lipohaemarthrosis should be present). Subtle, usually depression-type fractures may only be visible on X-ray as a subtle increase in sclerosis.

The proximal aspect of the tibia should not extend more than 5 mm past the lateral border of the femoral condyles. If extension of the tibial plateau occurs laterally, a split or depression-type fracture should be considered. CT imaging should be performed if a tibial plateau fracture is identified for full assessment of the fracture pattern.

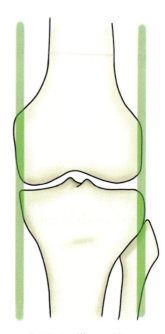

**Figure 3.18** An illustration demonstrating the normal alignment of the tibial plateau in relation to the femoral condyles.

## Classification of tibial plateau fractures (Schatzker classification)

The Schatzker classification system is one of the classification systems used to describe tibial plateau fractures. The Schatzker system describes the fracture types according to involvement of the medial or lateral aspect of the tibial plateau using the AP X-ray to help categorise the fractures pattern.

| **TABLE 3.1** Schatzker classification | |
|---|---|
| *Type I* | Fracture of the lateral tibial plateau (vertical split) with no depression or depression of less than 4 mm. Caused by axial loading with valgus force to the knee with associated medial soft-tissue injury. These are usually seen in younger patients with high bone quality. |
| *Type II* | Fracture of the lateral tibial plateau (vertical split) with depression. These are the most commonly seen in tibial plateau fractures. However, if the depression is subtle or difficult to appreciate on X-ray imaging, it can be mistaken for a Type I. Caused by valgus force to the knee with associated medial soft-tissue injury. |
| *Type III* | Focal depression fracture of the articular surface resulting from axial loading. Can be further subtyped according to the position of the depression; a lateral depression categorised as a Type IIIa and a central depression as a Type IIIb. These are uncommon and tend to be seen in osteoporotic patients. |
| *Type IV* | Fracture of the medial tibial plateau, depression of the fracture may or may not be present. Results from axial loading with varus forces, which are usually high energy. Associated with subluxation or dislocation of the knee joint and neurovascular and soft-tissue injury. |
| *Type V* | Fracture of both the lateral and medial tibial plateau (bicondylar fracture). Associated with high-energy mechanisms such as RTC with a combination of varus, valgus and axial loading forces. |
| *Type VI* | Fracture of the tibial plateau with a further fracture involving the proximal tibia with disassociation of the tibial metaphysis and diaphysis. The fracture involving the tibial plateau can cover a range of different fracture patterns. Associated with high-energy mechanisms with significant soft-tissue injury and are commonly open. |

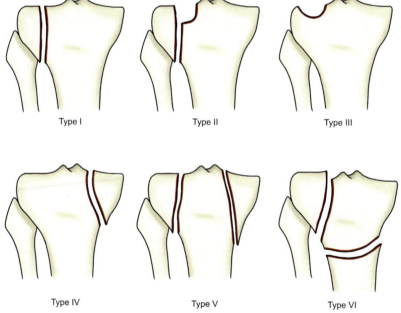

Type I    Type II    Type III

Type IV    Type V    Type VI

**Figure 3.19** Illustration of the Schatzker classification system of tibial plateau fractures.

## Distal femoral fractures

Mechanisms differ according to the patient's age. In younger patients, fractures of the distal femur occur due to high-energy trauma, which results in significant displacement of the fracture fragments. In older patients (especially osteoporotic females) fractures occur due to lower energy trauma such as a fall from standing height, with a lesser degree of fracture fragment displacement.

## Classification of distal femur fractures (AO classification)

The AO classification system uses three main classifications (extra-articular, partially articular and intra-articular) with further subcategories according to the degree of fracture comminution.

A: extra-articular – involving the metadiaphseal region

- **A1:** Simple fracture
- **A2:** Wedge fracture – usually seen in younger patients with high energy mechanisms.
- **A3:** Multi-fragmentation fracture – seen in high-energy trauma and low-energy mechanisms in osteoporotic patients

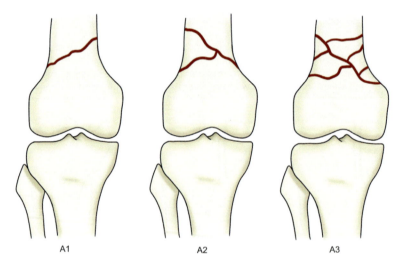

A1          A2          A3

**Figure 3.20** Illustration of the Type A fractures of the distal femur according to the AO classification system.

B: partially articular – vertical fractures involving the condyles

- **B1:** affects the lateral condyle (can be simple or comminuted)
- **B2:** affects the medial condyle (can be simple or comminuted)
- **B3:** anterior or posterior fracture, can affect one or both condyles. Anterior aspect fractures are often associated with patella dislocations.

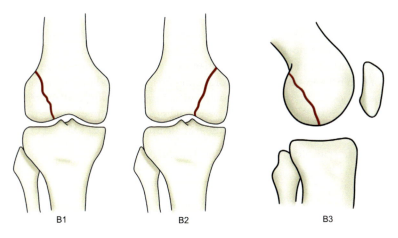

**Figure 3.21** Illustration of the Type B fractures of the distal femur according to the AO classification system.

## C: intra-articular

- C1: simple fractures involving both the metaphysis and articular surface
- C2: comminuted fracture involving the metaphysis with a simple fracture of the articular surface
- C3: comminuted fracture involving the metaphysis and the articular surface.

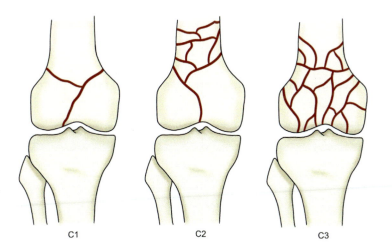

**Figure 3.22** Illustration of the Type C fractures of the distal femur according to the AO classification system.

## Degenerative disease of the knee

Osteoarthritis (OA) is the most common form of arthritis. This can lead to pain and reduced range of movement. The knee joint can be described using three compartments – the medial compartment (medial tibiofemoral joint), the lateral compartment (lateral tibiofemoral joint) and the patellofemoral compartment (patellofemoral joint – PFJ).

In the knee joint, the medial compartment is more commonly affected and will often demonstrate the most severe degenerative changes out of all three compartments. Grading of OA uses the following acronym: Radiographic appearance of OA = L.O.S.S:

- Loss of joint space (caused by cartilage thinning)
- Osteophyte formation
- Subchondral sclerosis
- Subchondral cyst formation.

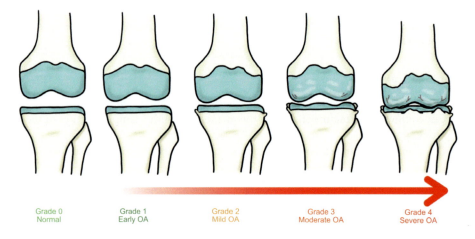

| Grade 0 | Grade 1 | Grade 2 | Grade 3 | Grade 4 |
| Normal | Early OA | Mild OA | Moderate OA | Severe OA |

**Figure 3.23** Illustration of the progression and grading of osteoarthritis in the knee joint.

| **TABLE 3.2** Grading osteoarthritis | |
| --- | --- |
| Grade 0 - Normal | No degenerative changes |
| Grade 1 – Early OA | Possible joint space narrowing<br>Subtle/early osteophyte formation |
| Grade 2 – Mild OA | Definite joint space narrowing<br>Definite osteophyte formation |
| Grade 3 – Moderate OA | Definite joint space narrowing<br>Multiple osteophytes<br>Subchondral sclerosis<br>Subtle deformity of the articular surfaces |
| Grade 4 – Severe OA | Marked joint space narrowing<br>Multiple large osteophytes<br>Significant subchondral sclerosis<br>Definite deformity of the articular surface |

# Systematic Assessment – Knee

## AABCS

- Anatomy and image quality
- Alignment
- Bones
- Cartilage
- Soft tissues

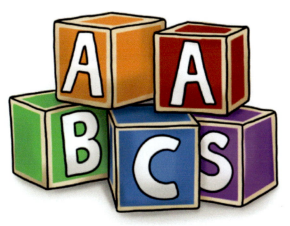

## Anatomy and image quality

Ensure the images are for the correct patient and are the most recent and up-to-date images. Is all the required anatomy demonstrated?

**Figure 3.24** AABCS building blocks.

Are the images of a good diagnostic quality? If not, consider why the images are of poor quality. This may be due to the technique used by the radiographer such as the exposures used or the patient positioning or it may be due to factors beyond the control of the radiographer such as patient body habitus or condition. External artefacts such as clothing, immobilisation aids or splints can mask anatomy or pathology.

## Alignment

**Alignment check for subluxation:** check the medial and lateral cortex of the tibial align with the corresponding femoral condyle. Disruption can indicate an acute injury or degenerative change.

**Check for dislocations:** these are usually obvious and associated with high-energy trauma. They are associated with ligamentous injury (so it is important to check for avulsion fractures). Patellae usually dislocate dorsally (due to the shallower femoral condyle); check the Insall-Salvati ratio. The patella may be sitting higher than normal (patella alta) due to contraction from the quadriceps. The skyline view demonstrates alignment but can be difficult to obtain in acute injury and is contraindicated if a patella fracture is suspected.

## Bones

The knee joint is made up of three long bones (Femur, Tibia and Fibula) and one sesamoid bone (Patella).

Assess the cortex and medulla of each bone individually.

Be aware of non-acute findings such as bipartite patella and osteochondral defects. However, always consider displacement of the bony fragment in trauma and Pellegrini-Stieda lesions.

Most knee injuries are associated with high-energy trauma, especially in younger patients. Therefore, also consider ligamentous and soft-tissue injury.

## Cartilage

Check the joint spaces are preserved. Degenerative changes should be noted as trauma can aggravate pain from these.

Check the joint spaces are clear. Opacity within joints may be caused by acute injury (an intra-articular loose body) or chronic degenerative changes (Chondrocalcinosis – which can cause acute pain).

Assess the articular surfaces, which should be smooth.

## Soft tissues

Soft tissues are a very important assessment region in the knee.

The joint capsule attaches to all the articular surfaces and then proximally towards the anterior femur and suprapatellar bursa.

Check all the soft-tissue fat planes and bursas to include:

- Infrapatellar bursa (Hoffa's fat pad)
- Suprapatellar bursa
- Suprapatellar fat pad.

**Lipohaemarthrosis:** two densities within the Suprapatellar bursa: fat (from bone marrow) and other fluid (usually blood – when trauma is suspected, but can be synovial fluid, pus, etc.). Presence of a lipohaemarthrosis can indicate an occult fracture.

**Effusion:** A uniform density within the suprapatellar region. Usually, a hyperdense fluid such as blood, synovial fluid, pus, etc. It can result from acute trauma or from chronic changes such as degenerative changes. However, the aetiology is not always known.

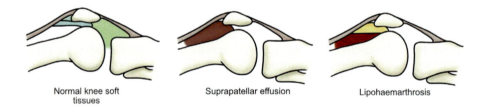

Normal knee soft tissues          Suprapatellar effusion          Lipohaemarthrosis

**Figure 3.25** The appearance of normal knee soft tissues, a suprapatellar effusion and a lipohaemarthrosis.

# Ankle Trauma

## Ottawa ankle rules

A clinical decision to help determine the need for diagnostic imaging. Patients that present with any of the following criteria require imaging according to the Ottawa rules:

- Bony tenderness at the tip of the posterior edge of the distal 6 cm of the tibia or fibula
- Bony tenderness at the medial malleolus
- Tenderness to the base of the fifth metatarsal
- Inability to weight bear for four steps (immediately or on admission to A&E).

## Ankle alignment

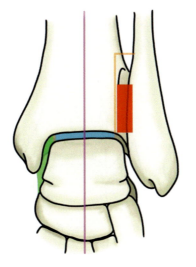

**Figure 3.26** Illustration of the normal alignment of the ankle joint, highlighting the tibiotalar line, ankle mortice and tibiofibular clear space.

Tibiotalar line: a line running from the middle of the tibial medulla should run through the centre of the talus on both the AP and the lateral image.

Ankle mortice: made up of three joint spaces. Assess the joint spaces on the AP image. All the joint spaces should be uniform.

- Medial aspect: between the medial malleolus to the medial aspect of the talus.
- Superior aspect: top of the talus to the medial aspect of the talus.
- Lateral aspect: between the distal tibial and fibula (not the talus). This is used in the assessment of the syndesmosis. Should be imposition of the tibia and fibula, if there is a clear joint space at this point. First, assess the patient positioning (is the image a true AP mortice X-ray) and then consider syndesmosis disruption/rupture.

The mortice joint is considered a ring bone structure – always check for a secondary fracture.

Tibiofibular clear space: measures 10 mm cranially from the tibial articular surface. At this level, the distance between the tibia and fibula should be approximately 6 mm. Widening can indicate interosseous ligament damage.

The ankle is supported by the capsule and ligaments. The medial ligaments are short and compact, making the medial aspect more stable than the lateral aspect and this contributes to inversion type injury. The attachment sites of the majority of these ligaments is at the distal tips of the malleolus. It is important to visualise these areas as it is a common site of avulsion type fractures.

## Weber Classification of ankle fractures

Fractures of the ankle are a very commonly seen injury and typically result from a twisting mechanism. Often seen in two distinct population groups: young active patients and in the elderly. Patients typically present with pain and an inability to weight bear. There is swelling around the joint with tenderness. When assessing patients for ankle injury, always ensure the proximal fibula is examined and findings documented, as associated proximal fibula fractures can occur. Patients with displaced fractures will present with deformity and possible soft-tissue injury. The Weber classification of ankle fractures is a system of classification which uses the fibula, relating to the levels of the fracture to the relationship to the ankle joint.

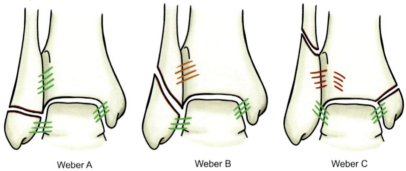

**Figure 3.27** Illustration of the Weber classification of ankle fractures.

### Weber A

Below the level of the syndesmosis, this transverse fracture of the distal fibula is occasionally associated with a fracture of the medial malleolus (if there is no fracture at the medial aspect the fracture is considered stable). Syndesmosis and deltoid ligaments are usually intact.

### Weber B

At the level of the syndesmosis – usually an oblique fracture of the distal fibula which is occasionally associated with medial injury (either involving the malleolus or deltoid ligament – widening of the medial joint space can indicate injury here). Syndesmosis is usually intact. There is variable stability, dependent on ligamentous involvement and ORIF may be indicated.

### Weber C

Above the syndesmosis and this may have an associated proximal fibula fracture (Maisonneuve fracture). There is syndesmosis disruption with tibiofibular joint space widening. Medial malleolus and deltoid ligament injury are often present. This is considered unstable and usually requires an ORIF.

> ### TIP
>
> Always consider a maisonneuve fracture when diagnosing a Weber C fracture on an ankle X-ray.

## Lauge-Hansen classification of ankle fractures

This classification can be used alongside the Weber classification system. The Lauge-Hansen system is based on mechanism of injury. Having a sound understanding of the mechanism can help predict the injury pattern that may occur. When used alongside the Weber classification, it will help to predict bone and/or ligamentous injury. In an ankle injury, fracture may not always be present. Therefore, always consider ligamentous injury.

### Weber A – described by Lauge-Hansen as adduction on a supinated foot

**Two-part injury pattern:**

1. Adduction causes tension on the lateral aspect of the ankle joint and this can cause rupture of the lateral ligaments or an avulsion type fracture of the lateral malleolus. The fracture is below the level of the syndesmosis and will be transverse in shape due to being an avulsion type injury.
2. Continued adduction can cause the medial aspect of the talus to impact on the medial malleolus. This fracture tends to be oblique or vertical in shape due to being a 'push off' type injury. However, it is uncommon for a Weber A type injury to reach stage 2 and a stage 2 is usually obvious and should be considered unstable (as the ankle is broken in two places). This is usually associated with high-energy trauma.

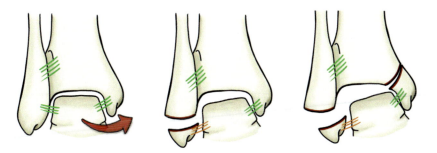

**Figure 3.28** Weber A fracture described using the Lauge-Hansen classification system.

### Weber B – described by Lauge-Hansen as exorotation on a supinated foot

**Four-part injury pattern:**

1. Rotation causes a rupture of the anterior aspect of the syndesmosis.
2. As rotation continues there is impaction of the talus on the fibula causing an oblique or vertical 'push off' type fracture of the fibula.

3. Following this, there will be a rupture of the posterior aspect of the syndesmosis or a fracture involving the posterior malleolus.
4. If the excoriation continues a transverse avulsion type fracture of the medial malleolus or a rupture of the medial ligaments will occur.

Fractures that reach stages 3 and 4 should be considered unstable.

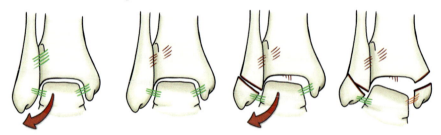

**Figure 3.29** Illustration of a Weber B fracture described using the Lauge-Hansen classification system.

## Weber C – described by Lauge-Hansen as exorotation on a pronated foot

**Four-part injury patten, usually associated with total rupture of the syndesmosis:**

1. Exorotation causes tension on the medial aspect of the joint, causing a transverse avulsion type fracture of the medial malleolus or ligamentous injury at the medial aspect.
2. Rupture of the anterior aspect of the syndesmosis.
3. Continuing exorotation causes impaction and a 'knock off' fracture of the fibula, which can be vertical or oblique shaped. Fracture is above the level of the syndesmosis.
4. Avulsion fracture of the posterior malleolus or rupture of the posterior aspect of the syndesmosis.

Fractures that reach stages 3 and 4 should be considered unstable.

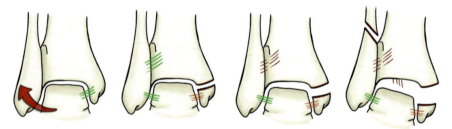

**Figure 3.30** Illustration of a Weber C fracture described using the Lauge-Hansen classification system.

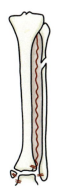

## Maisonneuve fracture

An unstable fracture of the ankle (Weber C), with an associated fracture of the proximal fibula. It may or may not have an associated lateral malleolus fracture.

This is an associated ligamentous injury, with distal tibiofibular syndesmosis and deltoid ligament injury with widening of the mortice joints and tear of the interosseous ligament.

If the ankle views demonstrate widening without a lateral malleolus fracture, clinical examination of the proximal fibula should be performed and findings documented. If appropriate, full-length tibia and fibula imaging should be considered to rule out a proximal fibula fracture.

**Figure 3.31** A Maisonneuve fracture.

## Tillaux fracture

A paediatric fracture involving the epiphyseal plate classified as a Salter-Harris type 2 fracture involving the distal tibial epiphysis.

This occurs in older children and adolescents. As the growth plate fuses from the medial aspect of the bone towards the lateral aspect, the anterior tibiofibular ligaments avulse the unfused part of the growth plate. In adults, the ligament is more likely to rupture.

It usually occurs as a result of external rotation of the ankle joint with supination. Patients will present with pain and tenderness (at the anterior/lateral aspect of the joint), swelling and an inability to weight bear.

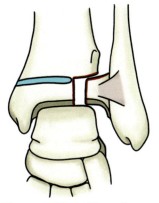

**Figure 3.32** A Tillaux fracture.

## Pilon fracture (tibial plafond fracture)

Fracture of the distal tibia with intra-articular involvement. Typically, this is as a result of high force mechanism injury involving axial loading, such as a fall from height or as the result of an RTC. This mechanism causes the talus to impact on the articular surface of the distal tibia resulting in a fracture.

Patients will present with pain, tenderness and an inability to weight bear. The ankle may be deformed with the risk of open fractures and associated soft-tissue and neurovascular injury.

Pilon fractures can be classified into three main types (Ruedi and Allgower classification system).

- **Type 1:** an undisplaced intra-articular fracture of the tibia
- **Type 2:** an intra-articular fracture of the tibia with significant displacement but minimal comminution
- **Type 3:** an intra-articular fracture of the tibia with severe displacement and comminution.

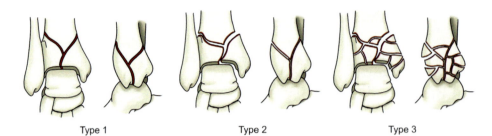

|                |                |                |
|:--------------:|:--------------:|:--------------:|
| Type 1         | Type 2         | Type 3         |

**Figure 3.33** Classification of Pilon fractures according to the Ruedi and Allgower classification system.

## Osteochondral defect of the talus

The term osteochondral defect is an umbrella term for a focal injury of the articular cartilage and underlying bone. An osteochondral lesion/fracture refers to an acute lesion, osteochondritis dissecans (OCD) usually refers to a chronic lesion.

Osteochondral lesion/fractures within the ankle most commonly involve the posteromedial or anterolateral aspect of the talar dome and is seen as a crescent-shaped fracture fragment.

## Talar neck fractures

Fractures of the talar neck account for the majority of talus fractures. These are most commonly caused by high-energy trauma, usually involving dorsiflexion with axial loading such as a fall onto a foot or during an RTC. Talar neck fractures are associated with further acute fractures.

Hawkins classification of talar neck fracture is:

- **Hawkins type 1:** undisplaced fracture. Blood supply is maintained with a low risk of avascular necrosis (AVN).
- **Hawkins type 2:** displaced fracture with subluxation/dislocation of the subtalar joint. Blood supply may be disrupted with approximately a 20–50% chance of AVN.
- **Hawkins type 3:** significantly displaced fracture with subluxation/dislocation of the subtalar joint. Blood supply is disrupted with approximately 20–100% chance of AVN.
- **Hawkins type 4:** significantly displaced fracture with subluxation/dislocation of the subtalar, tibiotalar and talonavicular joints. Often with associated fragmentation of the talus. Blood supply is disrupted with a poor prognosis and a very high risk of AVN.

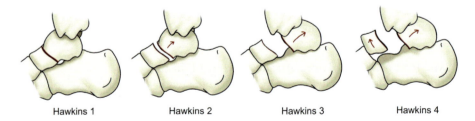

|              |              |              |              |
|:------------:|:------------:|:------------:|:------------:|
| Hawkins 1    | Hawkins 2    | Hawkins 3    | Hawkins 4    |

**Figure 3.34** Illustration of the classification of talar neck fractures according to the Hawkins classification system.

# Calcaneal Trauma

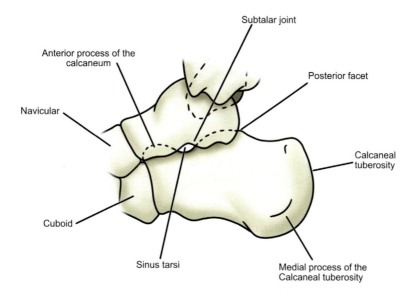

**Figure 3.35** Normal anatomy of the calcaneum.

The calcaneum is the most commonly fractured tarsal bone. Fractures in different parts of the calcaneum can be caused by different mechanisms. Axial loading caused by RTCs or a fall from height landing on the feet is a common mechanism of injury seen in calcaneal fractures and usually results in an intra-articular fracture, which is the most common type of calcaneal fracture. Fractures of the calcaneal tuberosity can be seen as a result of significant muscular contraction resulting in an avulsion fracture. Calcaneal stress fractures are commonly seen as a result of repetitive physical activity and usually occur within the posterosuperior aspect of the calcaneal body and will appear on X-ray as a vertical sclerotic line. Twisting injuries (commonly associated with ankle injury) can cause an avulsion fracture of the anterior process of the calcaneum as a result of strain on the bifurcate ligament. This area can be difficult to see on X-ray due to superimposition of the tarsal bones. However, an oblique foot X-ray will demonstrate this area well and it is important to check this area thoroughly in twisting type mechanisms.

Patients will present with pain, swelling and an inability to weight bear. Deformity with a widened heel and open wounds may also be present.

## Bohler's angle

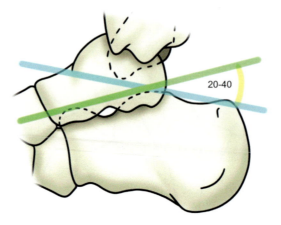

**Figure 3.36** An illustration demonstrating how to measure Bohler's angle.

The angle between two lines drawn from the anterior and posterior aspects of the calcaneum on the lateral view.

- **Line 1:** drawn from the superior aspect of the posterior tuberosity to the superior aspect of the posterior facet (blue line).
- **Line 2:** drawn from the superior aspect of the posterior facet to the anterior process (green line).

Bohler's angle should normally measure between 20°–40°. When the angle is reduced, it indicates a calcaneal fracture, however, a normal angle does not always exclude a fracture and Bohler's angle is considered to be unreliable in paediatric patients.

---

### TIP

Normal Bohler's angle does not always exclude fracture. Pursue further if clinical suspicion is one of injury.

---

# Foot Trauma

## Ottawa foot rules

A clinical decision tool to help determine the need for diagnostic imaging. Patients must present with pain in the midfoot plus any of the following criteria require imaging according to the Ottawa rules:

- Tenderness to the navicular.
- Tenderness to the base of the fifth metatarsal.
- Inability to weight bear for 4 steps (immediately or on admission to A&E).

## Midfoot articulations

The tarsometatarsal joints (TMTJs) should be assessed for dislocation or subluxation. Injury to this region can be subtle and easily missed.

To assess alignment lines should be drawn from the distal toes, through the metatarsals and into the tarsal bones. The lines should be straight when the joints are congruent.

- **Line 1:** Assessed on the DP view: the medial aspect of the second metatarsal should align with the medial aspect of the medial cuneiform.
- **Line 2:** Assessed on the oblique view: medial aspect of the third metatarsal should align with the medial aspect of the lateral cuneiform.
- **Line 3:** Assessed on the oblique view: medial aspect of the fourth metatarsal should align with the medial aspect of the cuboid.

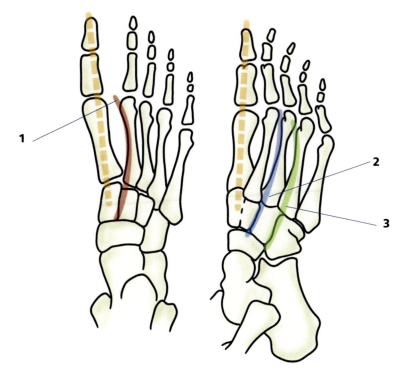

**Figure 3.37** An illustration demonstrating the normal appearance of the midfoot articulations.

## Lisfranc fracture dislocation

The most common type of dislocation involving the foot with dislocation of the tarsometatarsal joint with associated damage to the Lisfranc ligament. It can be caused by a range of mechanisms, such as crush or compression injury to the forefoot or axial loading and rotation on a plantarflexed foot (such as landing on toes after falling from height).

Patients will present with foot pain, specifically in the mid-foot region, swelling, pain and tenderness (especially over the TMTJs) and inability to weight bear.

Findings can be subtle on X-ray, so clinical assessment of the midfoot articulations is crucial. X-ray findings include:

- Bony fragments between the bases of the first and second metatarsals (fleck sign) and is associated with avulsion of the Lisfranc ligament.
- Widening of the joint between the bases of the first and second metatarsals.
- Displacement of the bases of the metatarsals with their corresponding tarsal bones – seen on the DP and oblique views.
- Dorsal displacement of the first and second metatarsals – seen on the lateral view.

Subtypes:

**Homolateral:** Lateral displacement of all the metatarsals, or displacement of the second to fifth metatarsals with the first metatarsal remaining congruent. Displacement is in one direction.

**Divergent:** Lateral displacement of the second to fifth metatarsals with medial displacement of the first metatarsal. Displacement is in opposite directions.

**Isolated:** This involves medial displacement of the first metatarsal with the remaining metatarsals staying in place.

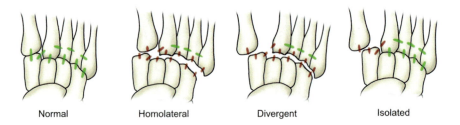

Normal        Homolateral        Divergent        Isolated

**Figure 3.38** An illustration demonstrating the different subtypes of Lisfranc fracture dislocations.

## Fifth metatarsal fractures

Avulsion fractures of the base of the fifth metatarsal are the most common type of injury in this region. Typically, a result of an inversion injury causing an avulsion of the insertion point of the peroneus brevis. When ankle X-rays are performed for inversion injury, always check the base of the fifth metatarsal, which should be visualised on the lateral ankle projection to ensure there is no avulsion fracture. Fractures should be transverse across the base of the metatarsal, vertical lucencies usually represent an unfused apophysis (in younger patients).

Jones fractures are extra-articular fractures of the base of the fifth metatarsal involving the junction of the metaphysis and the diaphysis.

Stress fractures are considered rare in the fifth metatarsal and usually occur within 1.5 cm of the metadiaphyseal region. They are most commonly seen in athletes or active patients or in individuals who have recently increased their activity levels.

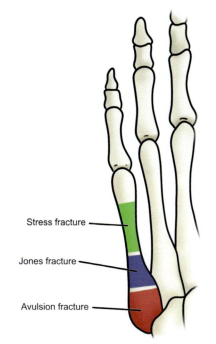

Stress fracture

Jones fracture

Avulsion fracture

**Figure 3.39** An illustration demonstrating the different positions within the fifth metatarsal of a stress fracture, a Jones fracture and an avulsion fracture.

## Metatarsal stress fractures

Fatigue fractures often seen in athletes, runners, soldiers, and patients who spend a lot of time on their feet and walking. More commonly seen in women and elderly patients.

Patients present with pain but minimal or no history of trauma. X-ray has poor sensitivity in the early stages however sensitivity increases as the fracture develops, due to formation of callus during the healing stages.

X-ray signs include:

- Periosteal reaction (however this may take up to 2 weeks to appear)
- Increased sclerosis
- Cortical thickening
- Subtle, un-displaced fracture line.

**TIP**

If there is high clinical concern for a stress fracture, but normal X-ray on initial presentation, commmence treatment then consider a follow-up X-ray to check for signs of healing.

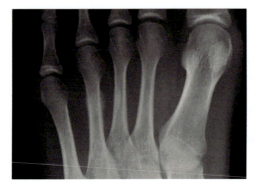

**Figure 3.40** X-ray demonstrating a healing stress fracture of the fourth metatarsal with callus formation seen. © 2022 University Hospitals of North Midlands NHS trust.

## Freiberg's disease/infarction

Osteochondrosis of the metatarsal head, typically affecting the second metatarsal but can also be seen in the heads of the third or fourth metatarsals.

Patients present with pain on weight bearing, swelling and tenderness. More commonly seen in young female patients (10–18 years old).

X-ray appearance:

- Flattening of the metatarsal head
- Widening of the metatarsophalangeal joint
- Cortical thickening
- Increased sclerosis
- Cystic appearance
- Fragmentation (in late stages).

## Kohler's disease

Childhood onset of osteonecrosis of the Navicular. Typically seen in children ages 4–6 years old with males more commonly affected. This is self-limiting with spontaneous reossification and reconstruction. However, this may take several years to complete full reossification.

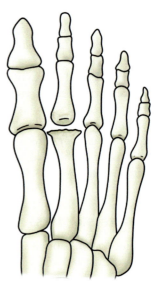

**Figure 3.41** An illustration demonstrating the appearance of Freiberg's disease.

Patients tend to be asymptomatic and Kohler's disease is identified as an incidental finding. Occasionally, the patient may present with pain, typically at the dorsal or medial aspect of the foot and a possible limp with a preference to weight bear on the lateral aspect of the foot.

X-ray appearance:

- Navicular appears flattened, thinned and sclerotic
- Sclerosis may be patchy in appearance
- Often associated with dorsal and medial swelling.

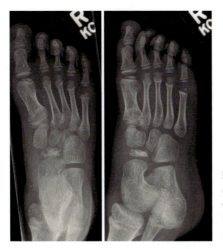

**Figure 3.42** An X-ray series demonstrating Kohler's disease. © 2022 University Hospitals of North Midlands NHS trust. All rights reserved.

## Systematic Assessment – Ankle

### AABCS

- Anatomy and image quality
- Alignment
- Bones
- Cartilage
- Soft tissues

### Anatomy and image quality

Ensure the images are for the correct patient and are the most recent and up-to-date images. Is all

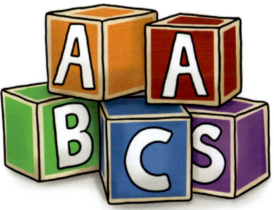

**Figure 3.43** AABCS building blocks.

the required anatomy demonstrated? Are the images of a good diagnostic quality? If not, consider why the images are of poor quality – it may be due to the technique used by the radiographer such as the exposures used or the patient positioning or, it may be due to factors beyond the control of the radiographer such as patient body habitus or condition. External artefacts such as clothing, immobilisation aids or splints can mask anatomy or pathology.

### Alignment

Check the tibiotalar line (running from the medulla of the tibial to the centre of the talus) in both AP and lateral views.

Check the three mortice joint spaces – medial, superior and lateral. Remember the mortice is considered a ring bone structure. If one injury is identified, check for a secondary injury. This can be ligamentous. Always consider if joint space narrowing is caused by trauma or degenerative changes.

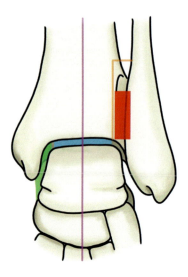

**Figure 3.44** Illustration of the normal alignment of the ankle joint, highlighting the tibiotalar line, ankle mortice and tibiofibular clear space.

## Bones

Consider the mechanism of injury to predict injury pattern.

Assess the cortex and medulla of each bone individually. There are lots of short bones in the ankle so assess the trabeculae thoroughly.

Check any adjacent or soft-tissue opacities and consider if these are avulsion injuries or accessory ossicles.

## Cartilage

Check that the joint spaces are preserved. If not, consider the patient's positioning, acute trauma or chronic degenerative changes.

Check the joint spaces are clear with smooth articular surfaces and check for subchondral fractures or osteochondral defects.

## Soft tissues

Soft tissues should closely follow the bony cortex; swelling is a good indicator of injury. Check for effusions. These will appear as a hyperdense region, usually at the anterior aspect of the joint. Hoffa's fat pad at the posterior aspect of the ankle should be visible and well defined. If there is loss of the normal appearance of Hoffa's fat pad, consider Achilles' Tendon disruption or rupture.

# Systematic Assessment – Foot

## AABCS

- Anatomy and image quality
- **Alignment**
- Bones
- Cartilage
- Soft tissues

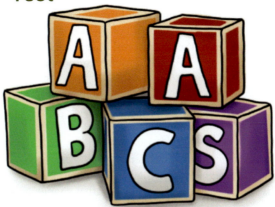

## Anatomy and image quality

Ensure the images are for the correct patient and are the most recent and up-to-date images. Is all

**Figure 3.45** AABCS building blocks.

the required anatomy demonstrated? Are the images of a good diagnostic quality? If not, consider why the images are of poor quality. It may be due to the technique used by the radiographer such as the exposures used or the patient positioning or it may be due to factors beyond the control of the radiographer such as patient body habitus or condition. External artefacts such as clothing, immobilisation aids or splints can mask anatomy or pathology.

## Alignment

The line running from this distal aspect of the toe, through the metatarsal and into the adjacent tarsal should be straight and congruent.

Check the TMTJ's:

- First metatarsal aligns with the medial cuneiform
- Second metatarsal aligns with the intermediate cuneiform
- Third metatarsal aligns with the lateral cuneiform
- Fourth and fifth metatarsal aligns with the cuboid.

Assess the Lisfranc region and alignment. On the DP image, the medial aspect of the second metatarsal should align with the lateral aspect of the intermediate cuneiform. On the oblique image, the medial aspect of the third metatarsal should align with the medial aspect of the lateral cuneiform and the medial aspect of the fourth metatarsal should align with the medial aspect of the cuboid.

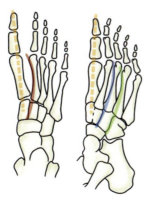

**Figure 3.46** An illustration demonstrating the normal appearance of the midfoot articulations.

## Bones

The forefoot is made up of long bones which are susceptible to stress fractures.

The midfoot is made up of short bones and is crowded with bony overlap but try and assess each of the seven tarsal bones individually.

Check any adjacent or soft-tissue opacities. Consider if these are an acute injury or accessory ossicles.

## Cartilage

Check that the joint spaces are preserved. If not, consider the patient's positioning, acute trauma or chronic degenerative changes.

Thoroughly assess the Lisfranc joint, as injury here can be very subtle. The first MTPJ is highly susceptible to degenerative change and it can demonstrate severe degenerative change even when the rest of the foot articulations are well preserved.

## Soft tissues

Soft tissues should closely follow the bony cortex – swelling is a good indicator of injury.

# Chapter 4

# Pelvis and Hip

**Overview**

Throughout the course of this chapter we aim to review the pelvis and hips.

Firstly we will review the normal anatomy of the pelvis, then work through common injuries and their radiographic appearance and identification. We will also look at developmental abnormalities, alongside degenerative change. Finally, we will cover a systematic review of all of these topics in a concise revision format.

## Anatomy of Pelvic Trauma

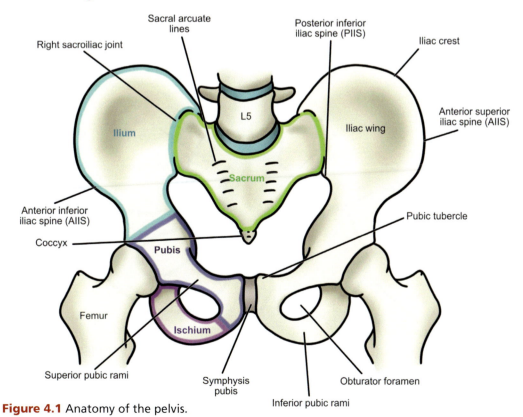

**Figure 4.1** Anatomy of the pelvis.

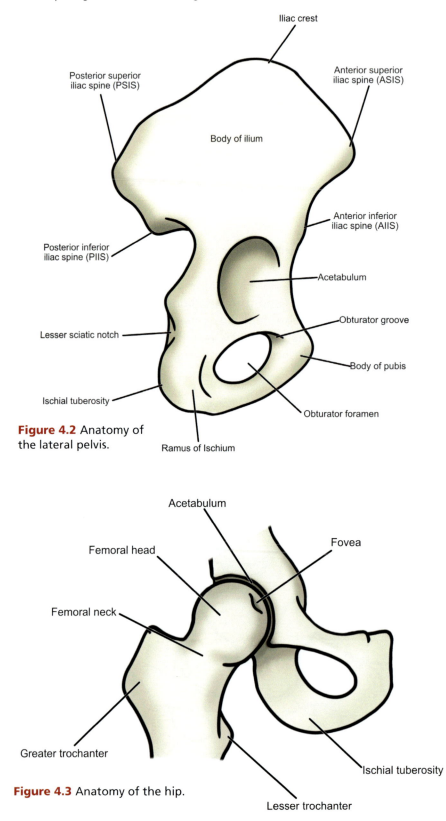

**Figure 4.2** Anatomy of the lateral pelvis.

**Figure 4.3** Anatomy of the hip.

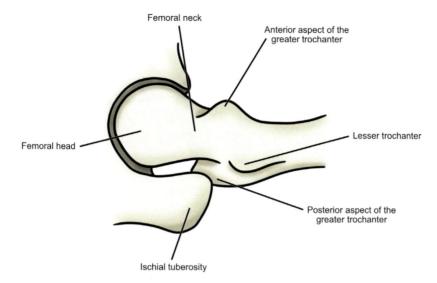

Femoral neck

Anterior aspect of the
greater trochanter

Femoral head

Lesser trochanter

Posterior aspect of the
greater trochanter

Ischial tuberosity

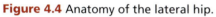
**Figure 4.4** Anatomy of the lateral hip.

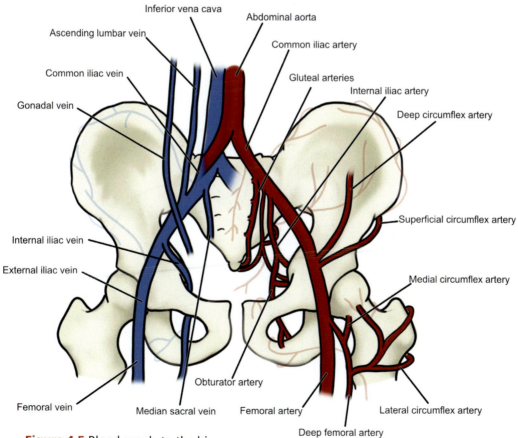

Inferior vena cava

Abdominal aorta

Ascending lumbar vein

Common iliac artery

Common iliac vein

Gluteal arteries

Internal iliac artery

Gonadal vein

Deep circumflex artery

Superficial circumflex artery

Internal iliac vein

External iliac vein

Medial circumflex artery

Femoral vein

Obturator artery

Median sacral vein

Femoral artery

Lateral circumflex artery

Deep femoral artery

**Figure 4.5** Blood supply to the hip
and pelvis.

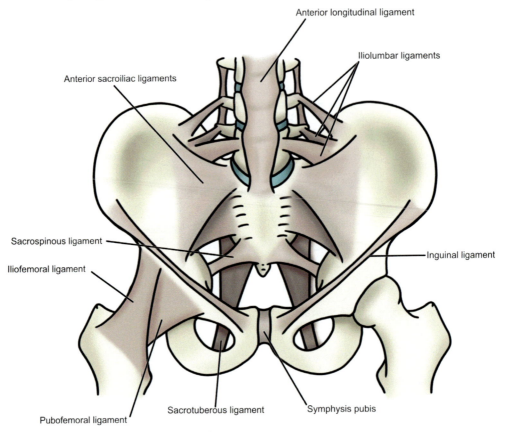

Anterior longitudinal ligament

Iliolumbar ligaments

Anterior sacroiliac ligaments

Sacrospinous ligament

Iliofemoral ligament

Inguinal ligament

Pubofemoral ligament

Sacrotuberous ligament

Symphysis pubis

**Figure 4.6** Pelvic ligaments – anterior aspect.

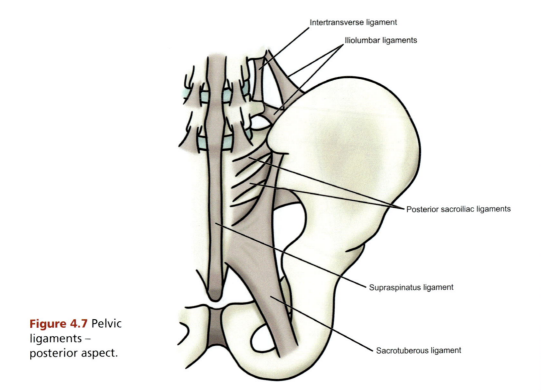

Intertransverse ligament

Iliolumbar ligaments

Posterior sacroiliac ligaments

Supraspinatus ligament

**Figure 4.7** Pelvic ligaments – posterior aspect.

Sacrotuberous ligament

# Pelvic Trauma

Pelvic fractures are relatively uncommon and are usually associated with high-energy trauma, such as road traffic collisions (RTCs) and falls from height. Due to the anatomy surrounding the pelvis and the proximity of blood vessels and organs, pelvic fractures are often associated with soft-tissue injury, such as haemorrhage (increased risk of bleeding due to close proximity of major blood vessels – commonly the internal iliac artery), bladder rupture, urethral rupture, etc.

As the pelvis is a ring structure, it is important to assess for secondary fractures/injury if a primary fracture is identified; however, if the secondary injury is soft tissues/ligamentous, it may not be evident on X-ray.

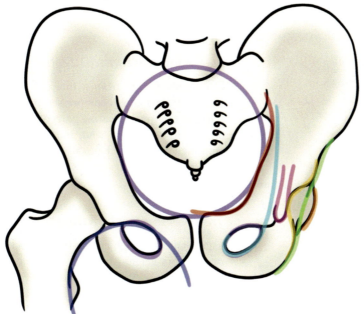

**Figure 4.8** Systematic review of the pelvis, highlighting the pelvic rings and assessment lines.

## Systematic review of the pelvis

There are three pelvic rings. Firstly, trace the main pelvic brim and then to two obturators. If there is disruption to the rings consider fracture, then look for a secondary fracture – the ring bone principle.

Next, check the pelvic lines:

- Shenton's line
- Anterior acetabular line
- Posterior acetabular line
- Acetabular roof
- Teardrop
- Iliopectineal line
- Ilioischial line.

**TIP**

Visualisation of all structures of the pelvis may be difficult in cases of major pelvic trauma due to overlying artifacts such as pelvis binders and traction splints (which may be applied in the pre-hospital environment). If appropriate, remove external artifacts prior to imaging.

## Pelvic fractures

The pelvis is considered a ring bone structure and, when there is a fracture in one part of the pelvis, there is often an associated further pelvic fracture or ligamentous injury. There are a number of different fracture patterns seen within the pelvis and they are often described as stable or unstable injuries. Stable pelvic fractures account for the majority of pelvic injury and involve only one break in the pelvic ring (however, these fracture fragments may be comminuted), the fracture usually demonstrates minimal displacement and is associated with low-energy mechanisms. Unstable pelvic fractures involve one or more breaks within the pelvic ring and are associated with a higher risk of significant bleeding and associated injury to the internal organs. Unstable pelvic fractures are associated with high-energy mechanisms.

## Stable pelvic fractures

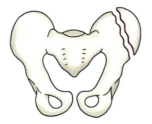

**Figure 4.9** Iliac wing fracture.

### Iliac wing fractures (Duverney fractures)

Commonly results from a direct blow to the iliac wing or from a lateral compressive force. Considered stable as the weight bearing parts of the pelvis remain intact. However, iliac wing fractures are associated with high-energy mechanisms and have associations with further injury such as soft-tissue and bowel injury (Figure 4.9).

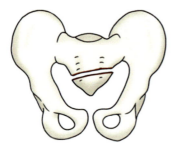

**Figure 4.10** Transverse sacral fracture.

### Transverse sacral fractures

Can result from high-energy trauma such as an RTC or fall from height (usually landing on feet) or low-energy trauma, especially in elderly patients. Patients will present with lower back pain and tenderness most pronounced at the sacral region. Sacral fractures are a common pelvic injury; however, they are often underdiagnosed as they can be difficult to appreciate on X-ray images (Figure 4.10).

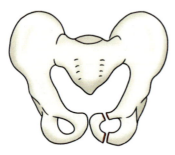

**Figure 4.11** Pubic rami fractures.

### Pubic rami fractures (unilateral or bilateral)

These are commonly seen in elderly patients resulting from a low-energy mechanism such as a fall from standing height (Figure 4.11).

These are usually treated conservatively and with mobilisation (once initial pain has subsided). There may, however, be associated vascular injury; the corona mortis is a common vascular variant (seen more commonly in females) which communicates between the obturator artery and the inferior epigastric artery, creating a link between the internal and external iliac arteries. It is located on the posterosuperior aspect of the superior pubic rami and is susceptible to injury following a pubic rami fracture and can lead to significant haemorrhage.

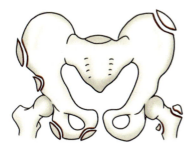

**Figure 4.12** Avulsion fracture.

## Avulsion fractures

These are commonly seen stable pelvic fractures, usually seen in young active patients (14–25-year-olds) and are associated with kicking sports (such as football) and gymnastics. Patients will present with pain, particularly on palpation of the avulsion site (Figure 4.12).

Avulsion sites and the muscles that cause them:

- Iliac crests = Abdominal oblique
- ASIS = Satorius
- AIIS = Rectus femoris
- Ischial tuberosity = Hamstrings
- Parasymphyseal pubis = Hip adductor
- Lesser trochanter = Iliopsoas
- Greater trochanter = Gluteus.

# Unstable pelvic fractures

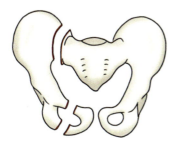

**Figure 4.13** Unilateral fracture involving the ischiopubic rami.

## Unilateral fractures involving the ischiopubic rami (Malgaigne fractures)

Usually, a vertical fracture involving one hemipelvis which is caused by vertical shear forces such as a fall from height landing on one foot. Patients will present with shortening of the leg on the affected side (Figure 4.13).

Fractures involve both the anterior and posterior aspect of the pelvis with fractures of the superior and inferior pubic rami and sacroiliac (SI) joint disruption most commonly seen, but can also involve fracture through the iliac or sacral body without SI joint disruption.

## Straddle fracture

Commonly caused by high energy vertical shear injury, such as fall from height and RTCs (commonly motorbike injury). Bilateral fracture of both the inferior and superior pubic rami with associated with injury of the genitourinary tract (Figure 4.14).

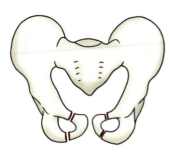

**Figure 4.14** Straddle fracture.

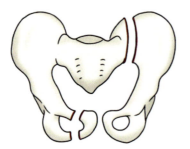

**Figure 4.15** Bucket handle fracture.

## Bucket handle fracture

Caused by anteroposterior compression forces resulting in a vertical fracture involving the anterior aspect of one hemipelvis – usually involving the superior and inferior pubic rami, and the posterior aspect of the opposite hemipelvis – involving the SI joint (Figure 4.15).

Not to be confused with a metaphyseal corner fracture (also known as a bucket handle fracture) seen in children.

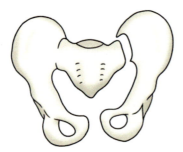

**Figure 4.16** Unilateral dislocation.

## Unilateral dislocation

A rare injury associated with high-energy mechanisms such as RTCs resulting in a dislocation of one SI joint with an associated dislocation of the symphysis pubis; associated fractures may also be present (Figure 4.16).

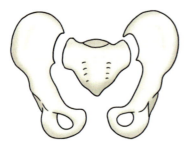

**Figure 4.17** Bilateral dislocation.

## Bilateral dislocation (Sprung pelvis)

Associated with high-energy mechanisms such as RTCs, motorbike accidents and fall from significant height causing anteroposterior compression or forced external rotation of the legs.

Results in dislocation of the symphysis pubis and both SI joints, with associated ligamentous and soft-tissue injury (Figure 4.17).

Some pelvic fracture classification systems can use different patterns of force applied to the pelvis to understand the fractures associated with those forces:

- **Anteroposterior compression:** Force applied to the pelvis from front-to-back or back-to-front. Causes fractures (usually vertically orientated) involving the pubic rami with disruption to the symphysis pubis and SI joints.
- **Lateral compression:** Force applied from the lateral aspect. Results in fractures involving the pubic rami, iliac wings as well as compression fractures of the sacrum. Central dislocations of the hip joints can also result from this force.
- **Vertical shear:** Force applied bottom-to-top, which can be applied to one or both sides of the pelvis (such as a fall from height landing on feet), usually causing vertical fractures involving the pubic rami, sacrum and iliac wings, and is associated with ligamentous injury.
- **Complex forces:** Will have at least two of the above forces applied to the pelvis at once.

# Hip Trauma

Hip fractures are commonly seen, especially in the elderly population. The increased incidence of hip fractures in the elderly can be linked to osteoporosis or reduced bone density in this population. The reduction in bone density can result in bony injury from low-force trauma, such as fall from body height, which is commonly seen in the elderly.

● Can be clinically and radiologically obvious – clinically, patients present with shortening and external rotation of the affected limb (however, if the fracture is un-displaced, this clinical presentation may not always be present).
● If the plain X-ray does not demonstrate a fracture (especially in osteoporotic patients) – further cross sectional imaging (CT or MRI) may be indicated if there is high clinical concern for an occult fracture, if pain persists, or if the patient fails to regain their normal mobility.

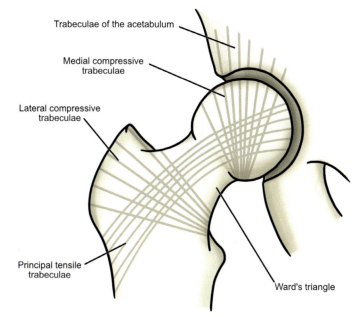

**Figure 4.18** Normal trabecular appearance within the proximal femur.

## Normal trabecular pattern

**Trabecular pattern:** A result of the supportive and connective tissues within the cancellous bone (concept of Wolff's law).

Wolff's law describes the ability of healthy bone to adapt to the demands and stresses placed on it – if more force is applied repeatedly to a specific area, the bony trabecula responds by adding additional support to that region in this hip which has a specific pattern.

**Shenton's line:** A smooth curved line drawn along the inferior border of the superior pubic rami and the inferomedial border of the femoral neck. This should be smooth and continuous. Interruption of the line can indicate fracture (or DDH). However, if the fracture is un-displaced, Shenton's line can remain intact.

## Fractures of the proximal femur

Fractures of the proximal femur can be classified into two main groups: intracapsular and extracapsular, with further subcategories of fracture within these two groups.

Intracapsular fractures occur within the head and the neck of the femur and can be classified as capital, subcapital, transcervical and basicervical. Intracapsular are associated with vascular injury due to the proximity of the vessels which supply blood to the femoral head. In cases of fracture with associated vascular injury, the risk of devascularisation and necrosis increases, which results in a higher risk of malunion and nonunion fractures. Intracapsular fractures involving the femoral head are rare and are often associated with dislocation, however, these carry less of a risk of vascular damage.

Extracapsular fractures occur within the region below the femoral neck called the trochanteric region. These fractures can be further subcategorised into intertrochanteric and subtrochanteric fractures. Extracapsular fractures carry less of a vascular risk than intracapsular fractures.

Fractures of the proximal femur are commonly seen in the older population and are associated with low-energy mechanisms, such as a fall from standing height. When seen in younger patients, they are associated with high-energy mechanisms such as an RTC. Patients will present with hip pain, pain on motion, an inability to straight leg raise and an inability to weight bear. If the fracture is displaced, the patient will present with shortening and external rotation of the affected limb with the possibility of obvious deformity.

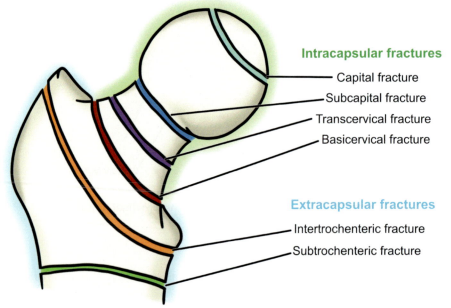

**Intracapsular fractures**

Capital fracture
Subcapital fracture
Transcervical fracture
Basicervical fracture

**Extracapsular fractures**

Intertrochenteric fracture
Subtrochenteric fracture

**Figure 4.19** Intracapsular and extracapsular fractures.

---

### TIP

If the initial X-ray does not demonstrate a fracture, cross-sectional imaging (CT or MRI) may be indicated if there is high clinical concern for an occult fracture, if pain persists, or if the patient fails to regain normal mobility.

# Garden classification of intracapsular neck fractures

The Garden classification system is commonly used to classify fractures of the femoral neck and is based on the position and displacement of the femoral neck before reduction using AP X-ray. Displacement is graded according to the position of the trabecular pattern, specifically focusing on the medial compressive trabeculae.

- **Garden I:** Stable, incomplete fracture. Some valgus displacement or impaction of the femoral head. Some valgus disruption of the trabeculae pattern.
- **Garden II:** Stable, un-displaced, complete subcapital fracture. No displacement of the trabeculae pattern.
- **Garden III:** Unstable, complete subcapital fracture. Valgus angulation of the femoral head. Valgus disruption of the trabeculae pattern.
- **Garden IV:** Unstable, complete subcapital fracture. Complete displacement of the femoral head.

This can be simplified into nondisplaced fractures (which include Garden I and Garden II) and displaced fractures (including Garden III and Garden IV).

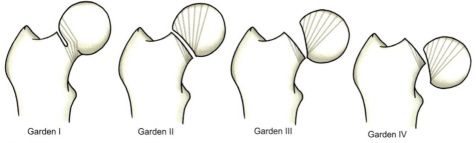

Garden I     Garden II     Garden III     Garden IV

**Figure 4.20** Garden classification.

## *Femoral shaft and neck angles*

Used in the evaluation of displacement of femoral neck fractures. The normal angle is between 125° and 135°. If the angle is reduced, this is classified as a varus deformity. If the angle is increased, it is classified as valgus deformity.

Varus = reduced
Valgus = long

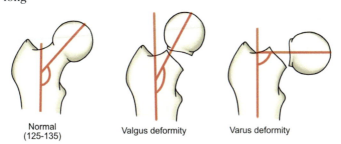

Normal
(125-135)     Valgus deformity     Varus deformity

**Figure 4.21** Different femoral neck angles.

## Hip dislocations

These are relatively rare, and usually associated with high-energy trauma such as RTCs; the hip joint is usually considered a very stable joint due to the associated muscular and ligamentous anatomy. Dislocations can be classified according to the position of the femoral head in relation to the acetabulum: posterior, anterior or central dislocation, with posterior dislocations being the most commonly seen type. Simple hip dislocations involve a dislocation with no associated fractures; dislocations with associated fractures are classified as complex.

Complications can include avascular necrosis, which is more commonly seen if the joint is not reduced within 24 hours, making swift diagnosis and reduction critical in order to reduce further complications.

Dislocation of a hip prosthesis following a total hip replacement or hemiarthroplasty is relatively common and can be as a result of very minor trauma. If a patient has a history of previous hip prothesis dislocation recurrence is common.

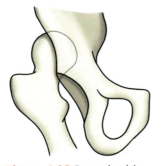

**Figure 4.22** Posterior hip dislocation.

### Posterior hip dislocations

This is the most common type of hip dislocation, accounting for 90% of hip dislocations. Typically, as a result of a high-energy mechanisms causing axial loading through to the femur with the hip flexed – commonly seen following RTCs where the knee collides with the dashboard. Patients will present with a shortened and rotated limb and AP X-rays will show the femoral head overlapping the posterior aspect of the acetabulum usually with internal rotation of the femur. It is important to thoroughly check the posterior aspect of the acetabulum for associated fractures.

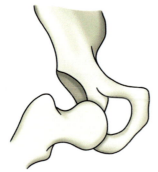

**Figure 4.23** Anterior hip dislocation.

### Anterior hip dislocations

Typically seen as a result of high-energy mechanisms with forced abduction and external rotation, commonly due to RTCs or falls from height. Patients will present with an externally rotated limb. AP X-rays will typically show the femoral head sitting in an inferomedial position to the acetabulum. Occasionally, the femoral head will be shown sitting in a superior position. However, this is rare.

### Central hip dislocations (protrusio)

These are rare and are typically seen as a result of a high-energy mechanism with associated comminuted fractures of the medial wall of the acetabulum. The femoral head will protrude into the pelvic cavity.

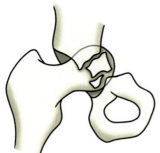

**Figure 4.24** Central hip dislocation (protrusio).

## Acetabular fractures

An uncommon injury which usually involves injury to the posterior aspect of the acetabulum. However, different fracture patterns can result in involvement of the ilium, ischium and pubis. Associated with high-energy trauma, especially when involving younger patients. Mechanisms can involve axial loading to the femur; such as a fall from height, an RTC or crush type injury.

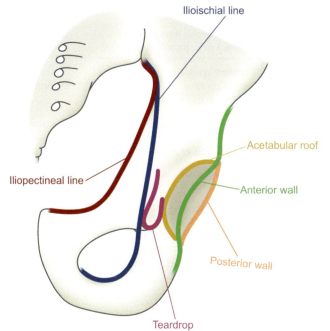

**Figure 4.25** Position of the acetabular assessment lines.

Initial radiographical assessment of the acetabulum can be done using plain film AP pelvic/ hip imaging by assessing the acetabular lines (six lines of Judet):

- anterior acetabular wall
- posterior acetabular wall
- acetabular roof
- iliopectineal line – checking for disruption of the anterior column
- ilioischial line – checking for disruption of the posterior column
- teardrop.

Each of these lines should be smooth with no steps or cortical breaches. When a fracture is identified, CT imaging is needed for full assessment of the fracture pattern and classification.

## Paediatric Hip and Pelvis

| TABLE 4.1 Differential diagnosis for children presenting with hip pain | | |
|---|---|---|
| Age | Common pathologies | Uncommon pathologies |
| Under 4 years | Transient synovitis<br>Osteomyelitis or septic arthritis<br>Juvenile idiopathic arthritis<br>Non-accidental injury (NAI)<br>Referred pain (usually from limb) | Leukaemia<br>Eosinophilic granuloma<br>Metastatic neuroblastoma |
| 4–10 | Transient synovitis<br>Perthes disease<br>Osteomyelitis or septic arthritis | Leukaemia<br>Ewing's sarcoma |
| 10–16 | Slipped upper femoral epiphysis<br>Avulsion fractures<br>Osteomyelitis or septic arthritis | Leukaemia<br>Osteoid osteoma<br>Ewing's sarcoma<br>Osteosarcoma |

### Transient synovitis (irritable hip)

A common cause of hip pain and limping in children caused by aseptic inflammation of the hip affecting the synovial lining. Pathogenesis is unknown however, there are links to recent viral infection such as respiratory infections. Patients usually present with a history of recent respiratory infection, pain for several days, with refusal to weight bear. The pain may resolve during the day and the patient may present with less pain but with a limp.

X-rays tend to be normal and non-specific and ultrasound can be used for the detection of a hip joint effusion and can be useful for a guided aspiration of the synovial fluid which may demonstrate slightly raised WBC and CRP.

Transient synovitis is self-limiting and can be treated with anti-inflammatory drugs and observation. However, transient synovitis presents with similar symptoms to septic arthritis of the hip, which can result in bone erosion and destruction, osteonecrosis and growth disturbance. The Kocher criteria can be used to help differentiate between transient synovitis and septic arthritis – if the patient presents with the following 4 criteria: an inability to weight bear, fever (greater than 38.5°C), raised WBC (greater than 12 000) and ESR (greater then 40 mm/h), the patient has a very high risk of septic arthritis and urgent treatment is required.

## Osteomyelitis

A relatively common, but severe condition. Most cases are caused by hematogenous spread (usually from a respiratory tract infection) with *Staphylococcus aureus* being the most common pathogen. Symptoms can be non-specific, but patients will present with pain, limp and refusal to weight bear. The joint may be warm, swollen and tender on examination. Infants may present with a fever and failure to thrive.

X-ray imaging does not demonstrate disease in the early stages. In children, osteomyelitis is more commonly seen in the metaphysis of the bone. Changes are usually seen on X-ray after 7 days, and these include aggressive periosteal reaction and reduced bone density. Osteopenia eventually leads to endosteal scalloping and loss of the bony trabeculae. However, X-ray is poor at seeing this in the early stages. In general, osteomyelitis must extend at least 1 cm and compromise at least 30–50% of the bone mineral content before it can be seen on plain film imaging.

## Slipped upper femoral epiphysis (SUFE)

Idiopathic Salter-Harris type I fracture involving the proximal femoral epiphysis is seen more commonly in males from the ages of 10 to 17 years; presents earlier in females (8 to 15 years) and obesity is considered a significant risk factor.

Patients present with no history of trauma with a long-standing history of pain, limp, leg length discrepancy or rotation and reduced range of motion.

AP and frog lateral X-rays are good for visualisation. On the AP view draw a line from the lateral aspect of the femoral neck. If this line fails to intersect the femoral epiphysis considered a SUFE. The frog lateral view demonstrates a SUFE better – the epiphysis usually slips posteriorly and medially.

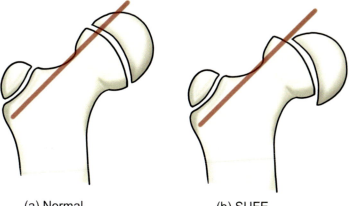

(a) Normal                              (b) SUFE

**Figure 4.26 (a)** Normal appearance of a paediatric hip and **(b)** a hip with a slipped upper femoral epiphysis.

## Avulsion fractures

This is relatively common in physically active adolescents and young adults – typically occurring in 14–25-year-olds and associated with sports such as gymnastics and kicking sports such as football. At this age, the tendons are typically stronger than the apophyses they are attached to. Strong muscle contractions will cause avulsion fracture rather than a tendon tear.

Patients present with sudden pain, usually following an action that will result in muscular contraction. On examination, there will be focal tenderness at the site of the avulsion.

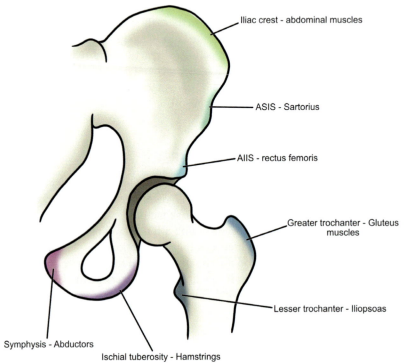

Iliac crest - abdominal muscles

ASIS - Sartorius

AIIS - rectus femoris

Greater trochanter - Gluteus muscles

Lesser trochanter - Iliopsoas

Symphysis - Abductors

Ischial tuberosity - Hamstrings

**Figure 4.27** Common sites of avulsion fractures.

Avulsion sites and the muscles that cause them:

- Iliac crests = abdominal oblique
- ASIS = Satorius
- AIIS = Rectus Femoris
- Ischial tuberosity = Hamstrings
- Parasymphyseal pubis = Hip adductor
- Lesser trochanter = Iliopsoas
- Greater trochanter = Gluteus.

# Developmental dysplasia of the hip (DDH)

Abnormal development of the hip leading to dysplasia, subluxation or dislocation. If detected and treated early, there is a high chance of normal hip development.

Before the age of 6 months, ultrasound is used to confirm diagnosis as the femoral head does not ossify until 4–6 months of age and will not be seen on X-ray imaging. X-rays are used to determine the relationship between the femoral head and acetabulum. Check for symmetry – check Shenton's lines, these should be smooth and the same on both sides (unless bilateral DDH). If there is disruption consider DDH.

The femoral head should sit within the acetabulum. DDH causes subluxation/dislocation – and the femoral head is smaller in DDH.

Hilgenreiner's line is a horizontal line running through the triradiate cartilage of both acetabulum and Perkin's line runs vertically from the lateral aspect of the acetabulum. A normal femoral head sits in the inferomedial aspect of the grid. The acetabular roof may be steeper in DDH (normal angle is 30°).

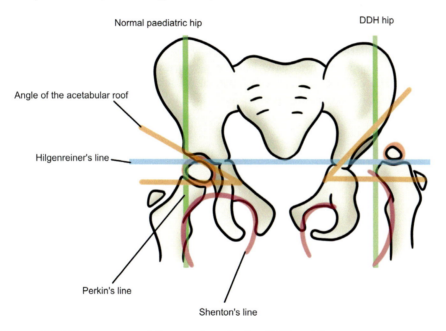

**Figure 4.28** The assessment lines and angles for DDH and its appearance on a normal pelvis (left) and a pelvis with DDH (right).

### Perthes disease

Idiopathic osteonecrosis of the femoral epiphysis affects males more than females (six times more likely) with no clear predisposing conditions. It is not caused by trauma and the changes differ from avascular necrosis caused by fracture or dislocation. Patients present with atraumatic pain (coincidental history of trauma may be present) or limp and blood tests usually come back normal.

The condition is self-limiting, however there are several distinct stages:

1. Devascularisation of the femoral epiphysis.
2. Collapse of the epiphysis.
3. Fragmentation.
4. Re-ossification and remodelling of the femoral epiphysis.

X-rays will be normal in the early stages. However, by the time the patient presents for X-ray changes may be seen. A subtle fracture line may be seen parallel to the hip's articular surface, known as the crescent sign. Joint effusions may be present and may cause wandering of medial joint space. The femoral epiphysis becomes dense and fragmented (first X-ray sign of necrosis). This is followed by collapse and flattening of the epiphysis (coxa plana) and enlargement of the femoral neck will follow (coxa magna).

Healing and remodelling eventually leads to a return to a normal appearance of the femoral head. If the collapse was severe or if there was late onset, then remodelling is likely to be incomplete and osteoarthritis is more likely later in life.

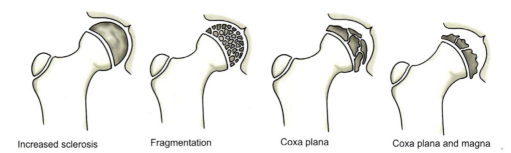

Increased sclerosis    Fragmentation    Coxa plana    Coxa plana and magna

**Figure 4.29** The four stages of Perthes disease.

## Degenerative Disease of the Hip

### Hip osteoarthritis

Osteoarthritis (OA) is the most common form of arthritis and can lead to pain and reduced range of movement in the affected hip joint. It can occur secondary to other causes such as trauma, avascular necrosis, Paget's disease, Perthes disease, DDH or SUFE – this is called secondary OA. Primary OA is related to degenerative 'wear and tear' with no other related causes.

Patients present with gradual onset of pain affecting the groin or anterior aspect of the hip. Pain can also often radiate to the knee and may even present as isolated knee pain. It becomes worse after activity, commonly associated with stiffness, sometimes limping and limited range of movement (internal rotation is usually the first movement affected).

Radiographic appearance of OA = L.O.S.S.

- Loss of joint space (caused by cartilage thinning)
- Osteophyte formation
- Subchondral sclerosis
- Subchondral cyst formation.

In the hip joint, as the articular cartilage is worn/thinned, the femoral head moves in relation to the acetabulum = migration. The femoral head can migrate in several directions such as superior, medial and axial (however axial migration is usually more commonly seen in inflammatory processes, such as rheumatoid arthritis).

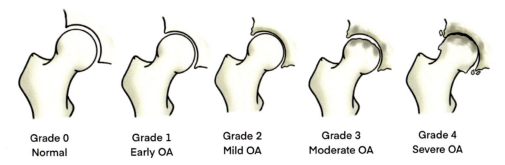

Grade 0
Normal

Grade 1
Early OA

Grade 2
Mild OA

Grade 3
Moderate OA

Grade 4
Severe OA

**Figure 4.30** Progression and upgrading of osteoarthritis in the hip joint.

| TABLE 4.2 | |
|---|---|
| **Grade 0: Normal** | No degenerative changes |
| **Grade 1: Early OA** | Possible joint space narrowing<br>Subtle/early osteophyte formation |
| **Grade 2: Mild OA** | Definite joint space narrowing<br>Definite osteophyte formation<br>Some sclerosis (especially in the acetabulum) |
| **Grade 3: Moderate OA** | Definite joint space narrowing<br>Multiple osteophytes<br>Subchondral sclerosis and subchondral cyst<br>Subtle deformity of the articular surfaces |
| **Grade 4: Severe OA** | Marked joint space narrowing – with bone on bone contact<br>Multiple large osteophytes<br>Significant subchondral sclerosis<br>Definite deformity of the articular surfaces of the femur and acetabulum |

## Femoacetabular impingement

There are two main types:

1. **CAM impingement:** caused by an abnormal femoral head/neck junction. Bony prominence at the anterosuperior aspect.
2. **Pincer impingement:** caused by abnormality of the acetabulum, with increased acetabular coverage.

Causes abnormal abutment of the femoral neck on the acetabulum, usually during the extremes of movement – specifically flexion and internal rotation, associated with pain. X-rays show loss of the normal contour of the femoral head / neck or acetabulum. MRI is indicated if there is associated labral tears or damage to the cartilage.

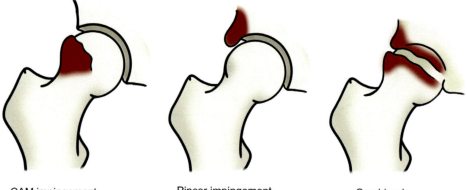

CAM impingement          Pincer impingement          Combined

**Figure 4.31** Types of femoacetabular impingement.

## Inflammatory arthritis of the hip

These are systemic conditions that are a result of underlying pathology, e.g. rheumatoid arthritis, ankylosing spondylitis, etc. Patients can present with pain in the groin, thigh, or buttock. This may cause a limp or reduced range of movement on examination. There are raised inflammatory markers such as ESR or CRP. Patients may be on disease-modifying drugs such as methotrexate to help slow disease progression. X-rays show joint space narrowing, osteopenia and articular erosions.

# Systematic Assessment – Pelvis and Hip

## AABCS

- Anatomy and image quality
- Alignment
- Bones
- Cartilage
- Soft tissues

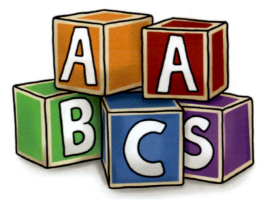

**Figure 4.32** AABCS building blocks.

## Anatomy and image quality

Ensure the images are for the correct patient and are the most recent and up-to-date images. Is all the required anatomy demonstrated? Are the images of a good diagnostic quality? If they are not, consider why the images are of poor quality – it may be due to the technique used by the radiographer such as the exposures used or the patient positioning; it may be due to factors beyond the control of the radiographer such as patient body habitus or condition. External artefacts such as clothing, immobilisation aids or splints can mask anatomy or pathology.

## Alignment

Check for **symmetry** between the two sides of the hemipelvis.

Is there a **dislocation** of the femoral head? Draw a line from the middle of the femoral neck passing through the centre of the femoral head. The line should pass through the centre of the acetabulum.

**Check Shenton's line:** Assess on the AP (feet in internal rotation). An arc drawn from the inferior/medial aspect of the femoral neck to the inferior aspect of the superior pubic rami = smooth continual arc with no acute angulation or buckling.

Check the six lines of Judet (focus on the acetabulum) which should be smooth with no angles/breaks.

1. Ilioischial line = posterior column.
2. Iliopectineal line = anterior column.
3. Acetabular roof = superior acetabulum (weightbearing region).
4. Anterior acetabular line = anterior wall of the acetabulum.
5. Posterior acetabular line = posterior wall of the acetabulum.
6. Teardrop.

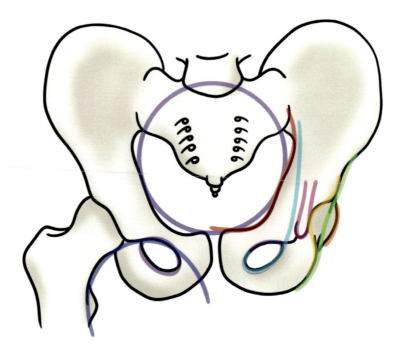

**Figure 4.33** Systematic review of the pelvis, highlighting the pelvic rings and assessment lines.

# Paediatric hips

**SUFE assessment:** Draw a line from the superior aspect of the femoral head, this should intersect the lateral aspect of the epiphysis.

**DDH assessment:** The patient may be too young for ossification of the femoral epiphysis. Use the position of the femur and apparent position of the femoral head to assess for dislocation.

## Bones

Check for **symmetry** – trace the outline of each hemipelvis and proximal femur.

Assess the **neck of femur** – common site for fracture: if fracture separates there will be a lucent line, if the fracture impacts it will show as a sclerotic line.

Check the muscular attachment sites for **avulsion fractures**.

Don't forget the sacrum – Check the SI joints and the arcuate lines (weak point of the sacrum). However, sacral fractures are easily missed on plain film imaging.

Check the bony matrix and trabecula – assess for lucency or sclerosis as the pelvis is a common site for metastatic deposits (plain film is poor for detecting metastatic deposits; MRI is gold standard) and be aware of overlying bowel gas.

## Cartilage

Hips are a common site for **degenerative change** and reduced joint space, osteophyte formation, subchondral cyst formation.

Check the **symphysis pubis**. This should have a close relationship with a joint space of around 1 cm.

## Soft tissues

Check the **fat pads** surrounding the hip – bowing can indicate joint effusion (can be difficult to assess if the exposure is poor) – gluteal, obturator and iliopsoas.

Check the **bladder** outline – is there any displacement? If plain film imaging is performed post contrast CT, there will likely be contrast contained within the bladder. This will make visualisation of the bladder easier but will obscure the sacrum.

> ## TIP
>
> Ostopenia can mask fractures – consider CT or MRI if there is high clinical concern.

# Chapter 5

# Spine

## Overview

This chapter begins with a review of the bony spinal anatomy within each of the four spinal regions, followed by an introduction to spinal review and alignment.

Common mechanisms of injury and common fracture patterns will be introduced with a concise systematic review of all spinal regions assessed. Finally, an initial overview of spinal deformity and chronic pathologies will be covered.

## Anatomy

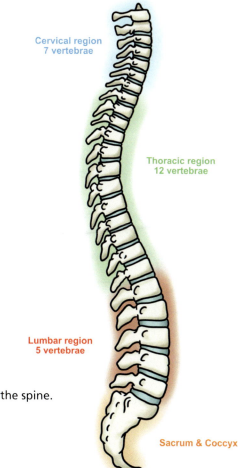

Cervical region
7 vertebrae

Thoracic region
12 vertebrae

Lumbar region
5 vertebrae

Sacrum & Coccyx

**Figure 5.1** Regions of the spine.

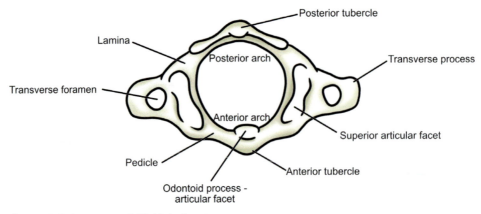

Figure 5.2 Anatomy of C1 (Atlas).

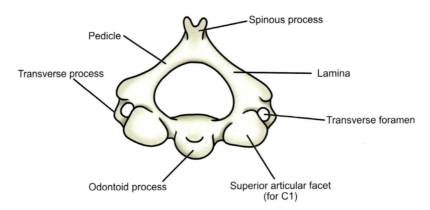

Figure 5.3 Anatomy of C2 (Axis).

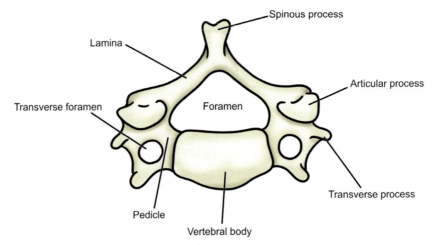

Figure 5.4 Anatomy of the C3–C7 vertebras.

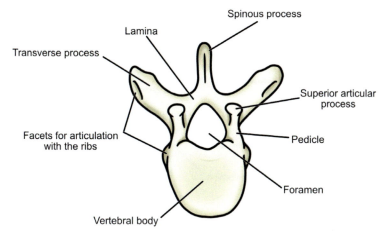

**Figure 5.5** Anatomy of the thoracic vertebral bodies.

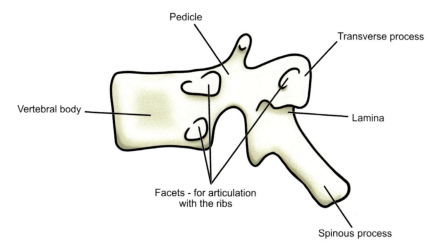

**Figure 5.6** Anatomy of thoracic vertebral bodies (lateral aspect).

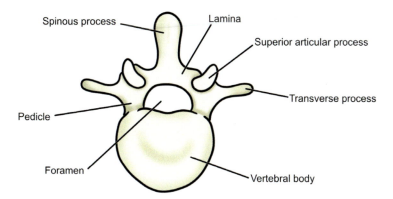

**Figure 5.7** Anatomy of the lumbar vertebral bodies.

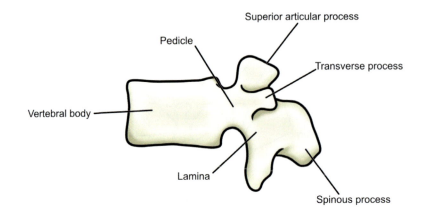

**Figure 5.8** The lumbar vertebral bodies (lateral aspect).

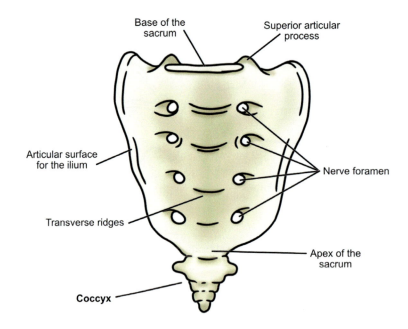

**Figure 5.9** Anatomy of the sacrum and coccyx.

# Cervical Spine Trauma

The cervical spine is susceptible to injury (both soft-tissue and bony) following trauma due to its high mobility and association with head injury.

Certain common mechanisms can result in specific fracture patterns:

- Spinal flexion = wedge fracture
- Spinal flexion followed by extension = subluxation or dislocation
- Spinal hyperextension = anterior ligament damage
- Forced extension followed by flexion = whiplash
- Vertical force through the spine = atlas/axis/odontoid fracture.

## Cervical spine assessment guide

### Four vertebral lines

- **Anterior vertebral line:** Anterior aspect of the vertebral bodies, should be smooth and continuous. Anterior osteophyte formation should be ignored when assessing alignment.
- **Posterior vertebral line:** Posterior aspect of the vertebral bodies, should again be smooth and continuous.
- **Spinolaminal line:** Spinal cord runs between the two posterior lines and offset of either of these lines is linked to spinal cord impingement.
- **Tips of the spinous process:** Should always be assessed as spinous process fractures are commonly missed.

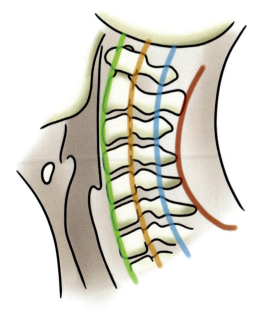

**Figure 5.10** The position of the four vertebral lines – anterior vertebral line (green), posterior vertebral line (orange), Spinolaminal line (blue), and spinous processes (red).

Pre-vertebral soft tissues are within the upper cervical levels (C1–C4). This should measure no more than 50% of a vertebral body width (on average 7 mm). In the lower cervical regions, (C5–C7) this should measure no more than 100% of a vertebral body width (on average 22 mm).

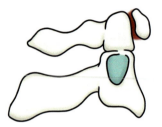

**Figure 5.11** The predental space (red) and Harris ring (blue).

**Predental space:** Distance from the Dens to the body of C1. In adults, this should measure 2–5 mm or less. In children, it is larger with 5 mm considered normal.

**Harris Ring:** This is a sclerotic ring projected over the base of the odontoid peg/C2. It may appear incomplete at the superior aspect, however, disruption of the anterior or posterior aspect can indicate a fracture.

## AP alignment

Check the spinous processes on the AP view. They should run in a straight line with the distances between the spinous processes remaining equal. Check the lateral margins of C1 align with the lateral margins of C2. The joint space surrounding the odontoid peg should be equal on either side.

This alignment can be distorted by patient positioning, so it is important to assess for patient rotation and the positioning of the patient's head. If the patient's head is positioned looking either slightly left or right, alignment of C1 and C2 can be distorted. When performing cervical-spine X-rays, the radiographer will strive to ensure the patient is as straight as possible. However, this may be difficult if the patient is immobilised.

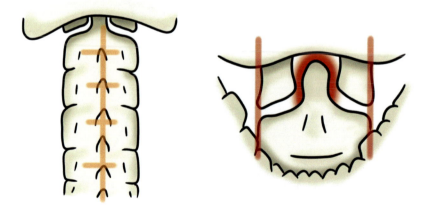

**Figure 5.12** Normal alignment of the spinous processes and the odontoid peg/lateral masses.

## Jefferson burst fracture

An unstable burst fracture of the C1 body involving the anterior and posterior arches with displacement of the fracture fragments. This typically occurs as a result of axial loading mechanisms such as diving headfirst into shallow water or as a result of a spear tackle in rugby. X-ray features:

- Widening of the body of C1 on the AP and lateral projections
- Reduction in the occiput/C1 distance and the C1/C2 interspinous distance
- Spinolaminal line disruption
- Lateral masses 'fall' laterally on the peg view
- May have an associated C2 fracture
- Pre-vertebral soft-tissue swelling.

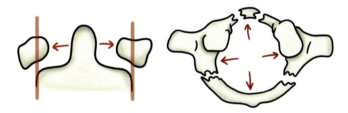

**Figure 5.13** The appearance of a Jefferson burst fracture.

## Odontoid peg fractures

These are typically seen as a result of high-energy mechanisms in younger patients, such as RTCs and as a result of low-energy mechanisms in elderly, osteoporotic patients, such as a fall from own height. Mechanisms tend to involve hyperextension which causes the bony ring of C2 to impact into the odontoid peg resulting in a fracture. Different levels of force and the quality of the bone can cause different degrees of fracture displacement and fracture patterns. Patients will present with neck pain, which is exaggerated with movement. Patients may support their own head manually and may also present with dysphagia (due to the presence of a haematoma).

The Anderson and D'Alonzo classification system can be used to describe fractures of the odontoid peg:

- **Type I:** A rare avulsion fracture (usually oblique shaped) involving the tip of the odontoid at the insertion of the alar ligament. Usually considered a stable fracture.
- **Type II:** Transverse fracture through the base of the odontoid, which may demonstrate comminution. Considered unstable with a risk of nonunion due to disruption of blood supply.
- **Type III:** Fracture of the base of the odontoid with extension of the fracture into the lateral masses. Usually considered a stable fracture with a good prognosis.

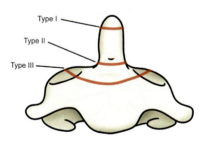

**Figure 5.14** The Anderson and D'Alonzo classification system of odontoid fractures.

## Clay shoveler's fracture

A rare but stable displaced oblique fracture of the spinous process within the lower cervical region (also seen in the upper thoracic region). This most commonly affects C7 but can also be seen from the levels of C6–T3.

This results from hyperflexion or direct trauma to the posterior aspect of the neck. Sudden muscular contraction can also result in an avulsion in this region. Patients will present with pain localised to the base of the neck or between the shoulder blades with reduced range of movement (particularly flexion and extension) and tenderness.

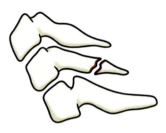

**Figure 5.15** A clay shovelers fracture.

## Hangman's fracture

A bilateral fracture of the C2 par intraarticularis, with associated anterior dislocation/subluxation of the C2 vertebral body in relation to C3 (traumatic spondylolisthesis). The fracture may extend anteriorly (disrupting the Harris ring) and may have further associated fractures of C1 and C3.

This is typically caused by severe hyperextension, for example, a hanging or an RTC and can be classified according to the mechanism of injury and displacement of the fracture as described by Levine and Edwards.

- **Type I:** A stable fracture caused by hyperextension and axial loading. The fracture will demonstrate minimal displacement of less than 3 mm with no angulation of the fracture fragments. The C2/C3 intervertebral disc space will be normal.
- **Type II:** An unstable fracture caused by hyperextension and axial loading followed by flexion. Results in a vertical fracture with more than 3 mm of anterior/posterior displacement but with angulation of the fracture site of 10° or less. The C2/C3 disc space is disrupted with associated injury to the posterior longitudinal ligament and there may be associated fractures involving C3.
- **Type IIa:** An unstable fracture caused by flexion and distraction. A horizontal or oblique-shaped fracture with significant angulation of the fracture site (greater than 10°) but with no anterior/posterior displacement.
- **Type III:** An unstable fracture caused by flexion and compression. Same fracture pattern to a type II fracture, with associated bilateral facet joint dislocations.

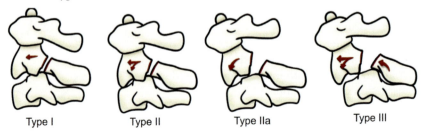

| Type I | Type II | Type IIa | Type III |

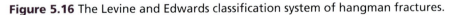

**Figure 5.16** The Levine and Edwards classification system of hangman fractures.

# Teardrop fracture

## Extension teardrop fracture

A rare fracture caused by forced extension of the neck resulting in an avulsion fracture of the anterior/inferior aspect of the vertebral body due to the insertion of the anterior longitudinal ligament (ALL). These fractures are more commonly seen in the upper cervical regions, usually around C2. Patients will present with neck pain but are usually neurologically intact. The fracture fragment is normally small, thin and triangular in shape and there may be widening of the anterior disc space with disruption of the anterior spinal line, but all other lines remain intact. Usually isolated to one spinal level and is considered stable in flexion and unstable in extension due to the disruption of the ALL.

## Flexion teardrop fracture

One of the most severe injuries of the c-spine caused by severe forced flexion with axial loading, such as an RTC resulting in severe deceleration or diving headfirst into shallow water. It is associated with ligamentous and spinal cord injury (anterior spinal cord syndrome and quadriplegia) and instability. Fractures are commonly seen in the mid-to-lower cervical region (C4–C6) and affect the anterior/inferior aspect of the vertebral body.

The fracture is comprised of several different bony and soft-tissue injuries: the anterior aspect of the vertebral body will demonstrate compression with an avulsion of the anterior longitudinal ligament (similar to an extension teardrop fracture). The fracture line will then extend towards the inferior endplate of the vertebral body. Further soft-tissue injuries will be seen at the posterior aspect of the spine with rupture of the posterior ligaments causing widening of the spinous processes. Posterior displacement of the vertebral body or fracture retropulsion will be seen, with subluxation/dislocation of the facet joints. This injury pattern results in compression of the spinal cord.

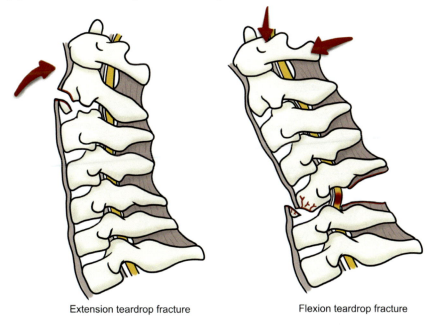

Extension teardrop fracture          Flexion teardrop fracture

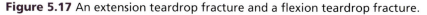

**Figure 5.17** An extension teardrop fracture and a flexion teardrop fracture.

## Facet joint injury

### *Facet joint subluxation and dislocation*

Facet joint dislocation is the anterior displacement of a vertebral body in relation to another with involvement of the facet joints. Facet joint dislocation is related to high-energy mechanisms in the young, such as RTCs and contact sports and low-energy mechanisms in the elderly. Mechanisms usually involve flexion with a distraction force. Patients will present with pain and numbness advancing to weakness and sensory changes with the progressive severity of injury.

Unilateral facet dislocations (usually involving the lower cervical spine) are often missed on X-ray imaging and are caused by flexion with rotational forces. This causes one of the facet joints to dislocate with associated soft-tissue injury involving the facet joint capsule and the posterior ligaments. The AP X-ray will show loss of alignment of the spinous processes with widening of the interspinous space. Subtle anterolisthesis may be seen however, if the anterior displacement of the vertebral body is significant, consider a bilateral facet dislocation.

Bilateral facet subluxations and dislocations occur as a result of flexion forces. Bilateral facet joint subluxations are known as "perched facets" and occur when flexion caused the superior facet joints to sublux and sit on top the superior articular facet of the vertebral body below. As the flexion forces progress the superior vertebral body will continue to move anteriorly causing the superior facet to move over the inferior facet and lock into place, giving this the name of "locked facets". Locked facets have associated injury to all the spinal ligaments with marked anterior displacement of the vertebral body and widening between the spinous processes. Locked facets are associated with significant neurological deficit. The superior aspect of the lower vertebral body may have an associated fracture and associated kyphosis.

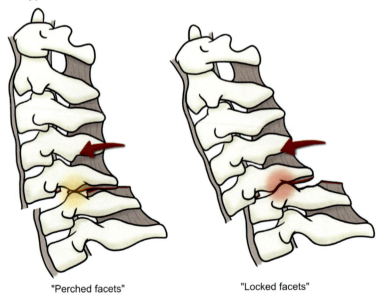

"Perched facets"        "Locked facets"

**Figure 5.18** Perched facets and locked facets.

# Thoracolumbar Spine Trauma

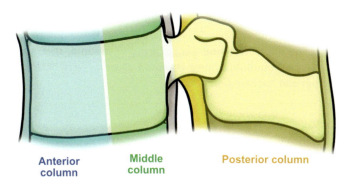

Anterior
column

Middle
column

Posterior column

**Figure 5.19** The three-column principle.

## Three-column principle

The vertebral body is divided into three vertically parallel columns:

- Anterior column = anterior longitudinal ligament, anterior 2/3's of the vertebral body and intervertebral disc (annulus fibrous)
- Middle column = posterior 1/3rd of the vertebral body and intervertebral disc
- Posterior column = everything posterior of the posterior longitudinal ligament – pedicles, facet joints, articular processes etc.

First developed to classify thoracolumbar injury but can also be used to classify lower cervical injury. The injury is considered stable if only one column is involved, considered unstable when two continuous columns (e.g. anterior and middle or middle and posterior) or if all three columns are affected.

## Anterior vertebral wedge fracture

Typically seen in elderly patients secondary to osteoporosis (osteoporotic vertebral compression fragility fractures) but can also result from higher energy trauma in younger patients. Hyperflexion injury to the vertebral body but can also be the result of axial loading. These fractures involve the anterior aspect of the vertebral body and are usually considered stable as only one column is affected. Patients will present with pain, usually at the level of the compression fracture and increased kyphosis.

Classifications (can be applied to wedge fractures in all spinal regions):

- **Grade 1 = Mild:** 20–25% reduction in the anterior vertebral body height
- **Grade 2 = Moderate:** 26–40% reduction in the anterior vertebral body height
- **Grade 3 = Severe:** Over 40% reduction in the anterior vertebral body height.

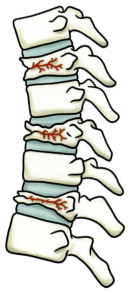

**Figure 5.20** A grade 1, grade 2 and grade 3 anterior vertebral wedge fracture.

### Vertebral plana

Also known as pancake vertebra or coin on edge vertebra. This is when the vertebral body loses its entire height, both anteriorly and posteriorly. However, the intervertebral disc space is relatively well preserved. There are a number of different mechanisms and pathologies that can cause vertebral plana including trauma, metastatic and myeloma deposits, eosinophilic granuloma (most common cause of vertebral plana in paediatric patients), infection and haemangioma.

### Burst fracture

A compression-type fracture resulting from high-energy mechanisms resulting in axial loading and flexion such as a fall from height or an RTC. This causes injury to the anterior and middle columns with associated retropulsion of the affected vertebral levels. The lower thoracic and upper lumbar regions are most commonly affected, with fractures involving only one vertebral level most commonly seen.

Patients will present with severe back pain which radiates into the flanks and limbs with altered sensation.

X-ray imaging will demonstrate loss of vertebral body height, usually most pronounced at the anterior aspect of the vertebral body with retropulsion of the posterior aspect of the vertebral body. The interpedicular distance on the AP X-ray view will be increased due to displacement of the fracture.

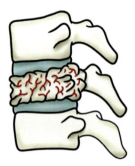

**Figure 5.21** Burst fracture.

### Chance fracture

Also known as seatbelt distraction injury, this results from hyperflexion-distraction forces often seen in RTCs because of forward flexion of the spine over a seatbelt-style restraint. During sudden deceleration, the region above the restraint is pushed forwards and distracts from the lower spinal region resulting in a fracture.

Chance fractures are considered unstable and involve all three spinal columns, usually an anterior wedge fracture with horizonal extension towards the posterior aspect of the vertebral body. Disruption of the facet joints and spinous processes will also be seen. Chance fractures have a high association with abdominal and gastrointestinal injury.

Patients will present with significant pain. Bruising at the anterior aspect of the abdomen following a hyperflexion-distraction force should raise suspicion of a Chance fracture.

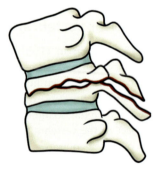

**Figure 5.22** Chance fracture.

## Spinal fracture dislocation

A rare but severe form of spinal column injury usually seen as a result of major, high-energy trauma, most commonly seen in motorcycle RTCs. Mechanism forces include acceleration followed by deceleration which causes forced hyperflexion and rotation which shears the spinal column.

It involves a fracture of the vertebral body (usually at the thoracolumbar junction) with an associated dislocation of the facet joints and disruption of the intervertebral disc. Spinal fracture dislocations are considered to be a highly unstable injury involving all three spinal columns, associated with a high risk of significant spinal cord injury.

Patients usually present with an accumulation of significant injuries which are usually life threatening, as a result of major trauma. Severe neurological injury is common, typically causing lower extremity weakness and/or decreased or lost sensation to the lower body, although depending on the level of injury this may also affect the upper limbs.

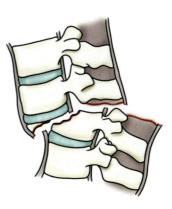

**Figure 5.23** Spinal fracture dislocation.

# Spondylolisthesis

A forward movement of the vertebral body (anteriolithesis), often due to a pars defect, a spondylolisthesis can occur at any vertebral level. However, it is most frequently seen within the lumbar spine at the level of L5/S1. The patient may or may not be symptomatic and when the patient presents with symptoms, they will usually describe pain at the affected level which is relieved with rest.

Lateral X-rays will demonstrate the position of the vertebral body, using the posterior vertebral line to assess for any displacement of the vertebral bodies. Displacement can be graded according to the amount of anterior displacement.
Myerding classification system:

- Grade 1 = offset less than 25%
- Grade 2 = offset between 26–50%
- Grade 3 = offset between 51–75%
- Grade 4 = offset between 76–100%
- Grade 5 = offset greater than 100% (spondyloptosis).

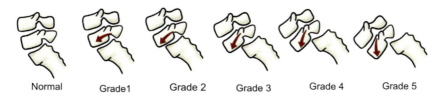

Normal    Grade1    Grade 2    Grade 3    Grade 4    Grade 5

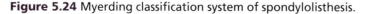

**Figure 5.24** Myerding classification system of spondylolisthesis.

## Pars interarticularis defect – spondylolysis

A bony defect affecting the area of the lamina between the facets called the pars interarticularis. It is thought to be a type of stress fracture caused by repetitive microtrauma. However, pars defects can occur as a result of high-energy trauma causing hyperextension. The majority of pars defects are seen at the level of L5 and can be bilateral, affecting both pars' regions or unilateral, affecting only one. When a pars defect is present, there is a high risk of spondylolisthesis.

Patients with non-traumatic pars defects are usually asymptomatic, however, some may present with lower back pain.

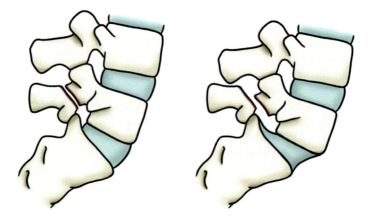

**Figure 5.25** Pars interarticularis defect and a pars interarticularis defect with an associated spondylolisthesis.

## Discitis

Infection of the intervertebral disc and adjacent vertebral endplates. In most cases, discitis is secondary to infections elsewhere in the body; the most common source being infections of the genitourinary tract but they can also be secondary to respiratory infections (e.g. Pneumonia), infections of the oral cavity, endocarditis etc.

In adults, discitis develops from an infection of the vertebral endplates (anteroinferior aspect) with spread into the intervertebral disc. In children, the intervertebral disc still vascularises, which allows for direct infection of the disc from any blood-borne agents. The most common pathogen is *Staphylococcus aureus*. Discitis can occur anywhere in the vertebral column, but it is most commonly seen in the lumbar region.

Patients present with a history of recent infection (UTI, pneumonia, etc.) with gradual onset of severe pain which is worsened with activity. Patients may also present with fever. X-ray isn't sensitive when demonstrating discitis, especially in the early stages. Soft-tissue swelling, followed by narrowing and destruction of the disc space, is the earliest plain film sign. Eventually, irregularity of the vertebral endplates will be seen with vertebral sclerosis if left untreated. MRI is considered the gold standard modality due to high sensitivity and specificity.

# Normal variants of the spine

## Accessory ossicles of the cervical spine

- **An accessory ossicle** of the anterior arch of the atlas, which is best visualised on the lateral c-spine projection as a well-defined density at the inferior aspect of the anterior arch.
- **Persistent ossiculum terminate** (Bergmann's ossicle) is a small well-defined corticated ossicle at the superior aspect of the tip of the dens.
- **Os odontoideum** is a well-corticated ossicle which is separated from the base of the odontoid process, usually around half the size of a normal dens.
- **A sesamoid ossicle** of the nuchal ligament is a common, well-defined oval opacity at the posterior aspect of the C5–C7 region, best visualised on lateral c-spine imaging.

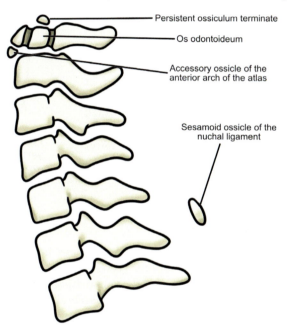

**Figure 5.26** The normal accessory ossicles commonly seen in the cervical spine.

## Common c-spine variants

- Pseudosubluxation of C2/C3 is commonly seen in children under 7 years of age and is more pronounced on flexion. The immature ligaments are lax and this is believed to cause this appearance. It is less commonly seen at C3/C4.
- Wedging of the anterior aspect of the C5 vertebral body is considered normal.
- In trauma:
  - Be aware that overlying anatomy can simulate fracture, e.g. overlying transverse processes.
  - Consider reasons for any altered relationship between the lateral masses in comparison to the odontoid peg (on the peg view). Can be caused by rotation of the head, which cannot be corrected if the patient is immobilised.

## Limbus vertebra

A common asymptomatic incidental spinal variant. It usually forms before the age of 18 but can be seen in adults. A defect of the anterior margin of the vertebral body, usually the anterosuperior aspect. Posterior limbus vertebra are less common but can cause nerve impingement. Radiologically appears as a well-corticated unfused secondary ossification centre and results from herniation of the intervertebral disc. It has a distinctive, well-corticated density with a sclerotic border, usually triangular in shape. Commonly seen in the lumbar region but can also be seen in the thoracic region.

## Schmorl's node

This is a herniation of the intervertebral disc through the vertebral endplate (more commonly seen at the inferior endplate), usually asymptomatic, but patients can present with pain. There is a small nodular concave lesion; some cases present with a sclerotic border. Commonly seen in the lower thoracic and lumbar regions, it is best visualised on CT but can be seen on plain film.

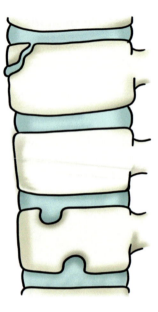

**Figure 5.27** A limbus vertebra and a Schmorl's node.

## Other spinal variants

- **Spina bifida occulta:**  A vertebral fusion defect found in 10–20% of the population. Appears in the midline as a defect of the posterior arch.
- **Butterfly vertebra:** Failure of fusion of the lateral aspect of the vertebral body.
- **A block vertebra** with complete fusion of the vertebral bodies.
- **Ring apophysis:** Secondary ossification centre of the vertebral endplate found in paediatric patients.

# Systematic Assessment – Spine

## AABCS

- Anatomy and image quality
- Alignment
- Bones
- Cartilage
- Soft tissues

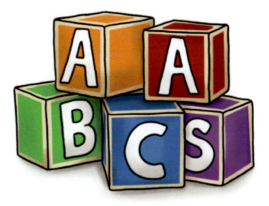

**Figure 5.28** AABCS building blocks.

## Anatomy and image quality

Ensure the images are for the correct patient and are the most recent and up-to-date images. Is all the required anatomy demonstrated? Are the images of a good diagnostic quality? If not, consider why the images are of poor quality. It may be due to the technique used by the radiographer such as the exposures used or the patient positioning or it may be due to factors beyond the control of the radiographer such as patient body habitus or condition. External artefacts such as clothing, immobilisation aids or splints can mask anatomy or pathology.

## Alignment

Using the lateral film…
Check the **four lines of alignment** (can be used in all spinal regions). All lines should be smooth and continuous with no sharp steps. Try to ignore degenerative changes such as osteophyte formation when assessing.

1. Anterior vertebral line = anterior aspect of the vertebral bodies
2. Posterior vertebral line = posterior aspect of the vertebral bodies
3. Spinolaminar line = junction of the spinous processes and lamina
4. Posterior spinal line = posterior tips of the spinous processes.

Using the AP film…
   Check the **lateral aspects of the vertebral bodies.** These should sit on top of each other with nothing protruding laterally (be aware of the effect of patient rotation!).
   Check the **alignment of the spinous processes.** These should run through the middle of the spine with equal distances between each spinous process. Malalignment can indicate facet dislocation/subluxation.
   Check the **distance between each pedicle.** The interpedicular distance will normally become slightly wider as you assess down the spine, but no sudden increase in distance should happen. This can indicate a burst fracture.

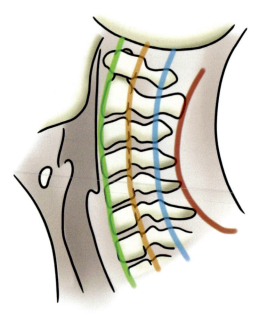

**Figure 5.29** The position of the four vertebral lines – anterior vertebral line (green), posterior vertebral line (orange), spinolaminal line (blue), and spinous processes (red).

## Bones

Assess the **shape and size of each vertebral body** (can be done on both the AP and the lateral view). Heights should be uniform within each spinal region.

Consider the normal shape. Is there any **wedging or angulation**? Check the superior and inferior endplates.

Be aware of **normal variants** and **secondary ossification centres**.

## Cartilage

Check the **intervertebral disc spaces**. These should be uniform and equal.

**C-Spine.** Check the **pre-dental space** (lateral image) between the C2 dens and the anterior aspect of C1, should be **3 mm** or less in adults and **5 mm** or less in children. Widening can indicate injury (possible ligamentous), but can also be caused by rheumatoid arthritis.

## Soft tissues

**C-spine – prevertebral soft tissues** (lateral view). At the level of C1–C4 should be no more than half the vertebral body width; at the level of C4–C7 should be no more than a whole vertebral body width. It should be uniform with no bulging. This can indicate inflammation or haematoma which may indicate acute trauma.

**T-spine – paravertebral line** (AP view) can be hard to visualise due to overlying anatomy. It should run to the left lateral aspect of the vertebral column and should be smooth, bulging can indicate inflammation or haematoma associated with acute trauma.

# Ankylosing Spondylitis

Ankylosing spondylitis is characterised by inflammation affecting the SI joints and the spine (but can also affect other regions of the body). There is a strong association with the *HLA-B27* gene. The *HLA-B27* gene is believed to be present in a small number of the Caucasian population. However, of the individuals carrying this gene, a significant percentage will go on to develop ankylosing spondylitis.

Typical patients are young males, presenting with long-standing back pain which may wake them during the night (Ibuprofen provides slight pain relief). Patients will have a stiff back with reduced lordosis and reduced lateral flexion movement. They will be *HLA-B27* gene positive.

## Radiographic appearance

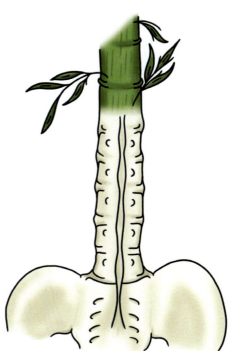

**Figure 5.30** The 'bamboo spine' appearance of ankylosing spondylitis.

- **Sacroilitis:** Usually bilateral and symmetrical, affecting the lower third of the sacroiliac joints first particularly at the iliac aspect. Loss of joint margins, erosions, joint space widening and sclerosis can all be seen. As the disease progresses, the joint spaces become less defined and eventually ankylose.
- **Spondylitis** with associated erosions and new bone formation. New bone formation along the anterior aspect of the spine causes a squared appearance – early appearance can be seen on the lateral image; erosions are seen at the superior and inferior vertebral endplates (Romanus lesions), reactive sclerosis/healing due to these erosions develops causing an appearance known as the 'shiny corner sign', and eventually, the vertebral bodies appear squared before becoming fully ankylosed.
- **Soft-tissue calcifications:** Ligamentous calcification can occur, for example, calcification of the posterior aspect of the SI joints and posterior interspinous ligament can cause an appearance known as the 'dagger sign'.
- Reduced bone density.

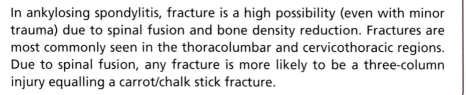

## TIP

In ankylosing spondylitis, fracture is a high possibility (even with minor trauma) due to spinal fusion and bone density reduction. Fractures are most commonly seen in the thoracolumbar and cervicothoracic regions. Due to spinal fusion, any fracture is more likely to be a three-column injury equalling a carrot/chalk stick fracture.

## Distribution

Distribution always involves the axial skeleton, usually affecting the spine and the SI joints. Sometimes involves medium/large joints such as the hips and shoulders. Inflammation of tendon and ligamentous insertion joints are commonly seen at the SI joints, iliac crests, gluteal and tibial tuberosities.

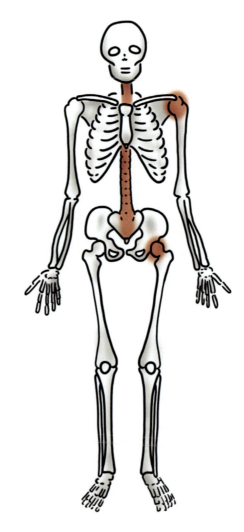

**Figure 5.31** Distribution of ankylosing spondylitis.

# Diffuse Idiopathic Skeletal Hyperostosis

Diffuse idiopathic skeletal hyperostosis (DISH) is also known as Forestier's disease. This is a common condition (usually affecting the elderly) and is characterised by bony proliferations at the insertion points of the ligaments and tendons within the spine. Usually an incidental finding, however patients may sometimes present with back pain and stiffness, with this stiffness usually being worse in the mornings. The imaging appearance is usually more severe than the clinical presentation.

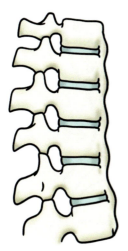

## Radiographic appearance

Very strict radiographic diagnosis criteria.

- Flowing anterior ossification – flowing ossification of the ALL which must involve at least four continuous vertebral levels.
- Bone density is usually normal.
- Intervertebral disc spaces are preserved with no narrowing.
- No involvement of the SI joints (no ankylosis or erosions) with any involvement of the SI joints excluding DISH as a differential.
- No significant facet joint arthropathy.
- Can cause enthesopathy elsewhere, e.g. the pelvis (iliac crests, ischial tuberosities, iliolumbar ligaments), Achilles tendon, triceps tendon.

**Figure 5.32** The radiographic appearance of DISH.

## Distribution

Usually seen within the thoracic region (most commonly the lower thoracic region). However, it is also seen, but less commonly, within the cervical and lumbar regions. The left lateral aspect within the thoracic region may not demonstrate ossification due to the close relation to the pulsation of the aorta.

Plain film imaging is considered the best modality for diagnosis, with CT considered optimal following a complication, such as trauma; due to fusion of the anterior aspect transverse fractures can result from minor trauma. Fractures can be non-displaced and may only be seen using CT imaging.

As DISH is usually an incidental finding, treatment isn't usually required. Analgesics (NSAIDs) can be used to relieve pain and stiffness. Some cases may require osteophyte resection if symptoms develop due to mass effect (especially in the neck). Large osteophytes can compress on several structures, such as the inferior vena cava and the oesophagus.

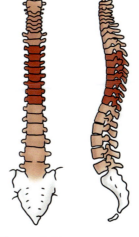

**Figure 5.33** An illustration showing the distribution of DISH.

# Spinal deformity

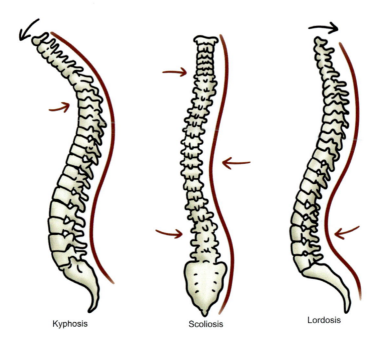

Kyphosis          Scoliosis          Lordosis

**Figure 5.34** The three main types of spinal deformity – kyphosis, scoliosis and lordosis.

## Kyphosis

A term used to describe a sagittal curvature, usually seen in the thoracic region, with an angle greater than 60° considered abnormal. Increased kyphosis is related to osteoporosis, spondyloarthropathies (such as ankylosing spondylitis, psoriatic arthritis, etc), trauma resulting in vertebral fracture and Scheuermann disease.

**Gibbus deformity:** The anterior collapse of one or more vertebral bodies, causing a sharply angled kyphosis. There are several different causes broadly split into congenital causes, such as achondroplasia or cretinism, and acquired causes, such as compression fracture, vertebral plana and infection such as osteomyelitis, discitis or spinal tuberculosis (Pott disease).

**Scheuermann disease:** Also known as juvenile kyphosis, this is relatively common, seen affecting approximately 5% of the population. Patients usually present around adolescence, typically with tiredness, stiffness, pain (usually made worse by bending, twisting or arching), limited flexibility and tight hamstrings. Results in an increased kyphosis in the thoracic/thoracolumbar region. The thoracic region is most commonly affected. Diagnosis is usually made on plain film imaging with increased spinal kyphosis (over 40° in the thoracic region and over 30° in the thoracolumbar region considered abnormal. Three or more adjacent vertebral bodies demonstrate wedging with endplate irregularity or disc space narrowing possibly seen. Also associated with Schmorl's nodes, limbus vertebra, scoliosis and spondylolisthesis.

## Lordosis

A term used to describe an abnormal anterior curvature, usually seen in the cervical and lumbar regions. Both of these regions usually demonstrate a lordotic appearance and increased lordosis in these regions is also known as hyper-lordosis. This can be the result of poor posture, obesity, spinal region or weakness of the core muscles. Hyper-lordosis can also be seen in pregnancy as the body adjusts to additional weight.

## Scoliosis

A lateral spinal curvature (with a cobb angle of more than 10°), can be caused by underlying congenital or developmental abnormalities but, in most cases, it is idiopathic. It can consist of one or more lateral curvatures but can also affect the spine in all three dimensions and may have a rotational element.

   The severity and progression of scoliosis can be measured using the Cobb angle. This is a measurement made from the top of the superior end vertebra to the bottom of the inferior end vertebra. In order to correctly measure the cobb angle, a two-key vertebral levels must be identified – the end vertebras. These are the vertebral bodies that demonstrate the most tilt in the curvature. A line is drawn from the endplates of each vertebral body and the angle at which they intersect is the Cobb angle. If the curvature is less pronounced, these lines may not intersect so an additional two lines plotted at right angles can be used to identify the Cobb angle, which is at the point that these two additional lines intersect.

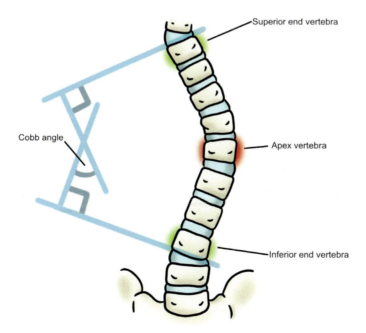

**Figure 5.35** Measurements for scoliosis.

Further key vertebral levels include the apex vertebra, which is the vertebral body most laterally deviated from the midline and represents the centre of the scoliosis apex. The neutral vertebra are the vertebral levels that show no visible rotation (both pedicles will be visible and equidistant from the midline of the vertebral body). This vertebral level is usually the best level to stop a surgical spinal fixation.

# Chapter 6

# Facial Bones

## Overview

This chapter will cover the facial bones and mandible. An overview of the region's anatomy will be followed by an introduction to facial trauma and the commonly associated injury patterns.

An introduction to the system of X-ray review will help establish a systematic search pattern when assessing X-rays of the face. Following this, we will cover mandible injury with an introduction to conditions which affect the teeth. Paediatric trauma to the face and skull will be introduced. Finally, a review of the regional systematic reviews will follow using a concise revision format.

## Anatomy

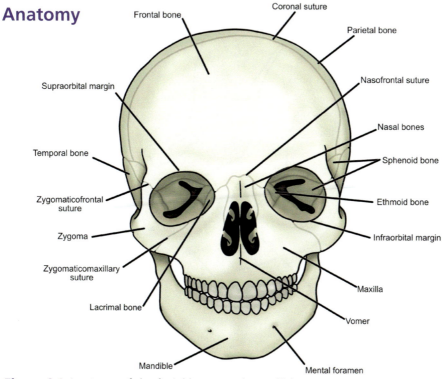

**Figure 6.1** Anatomy of the facial bones and mandible.

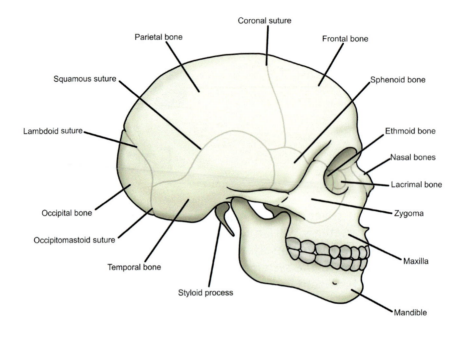

**Figure 6.2** Anatomy of the cranial and facial bones.

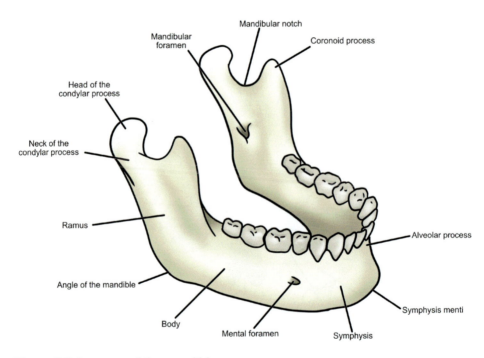

**Figure 6.3** Anatomy of the mandible.

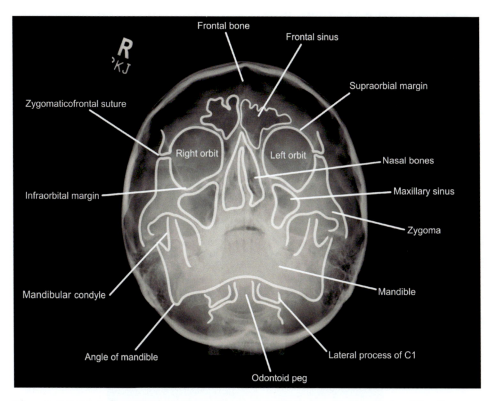

Frontal bone
Frontal sinus
R
?KJ
Supraorbial margin
Zygomaticofrontal suture
Right orbit
Left orbit
Nasal bones
Infraorbital margin
Maxillary sinus
Zygoma
Mandibular condyle
Mandible
Angle of mandible
Lateral process of C1
Odontoid peg

**Figure 6.4** A labelled OM facial bone X-ray. © 2022 University Hospitals of North Midlands NHS Trust.

## Facial Trauma

Facial bone fracture and injury is often associated with a direct blow to the face, such as in suspected assaults, RTCs and falls. When clinically assessing the face, remember to assess the patient's vision, completing a full range of movement of the eyes checking for diplopia and assess the dentition and alignment of the teeth. Clear documentation of both clinical and radiological findings will always be required from a medicolegal point of view.

Assessment of facial bone X-rays can be difficult due to the complex superimposed structures within the facial and cranial regions. Injury patterns to the face tend to follow several recognised patterns and systematic review aids have been created in order to fully assess facial bone X-rays to assess for injury.

Facial bone X-rays are slightly different to normal X-ray images in that the two views the radiographer produces are not perpendicular. Standard facial bone X-rays are performed with different caudal angulation; the first view is the Occipitomental (OM) view which is performed with no angle and with the primary X-ray beam perpendicular to the X-ray detector. The OM is the best view for the assessment of fluid levels within the sinuses. The second view is the Occipitomental 30° (OM30) view which is performed with a 30° caudal angulation in relation to the X-ray detector.

> **TIP**
>
> Remember to use lines and symmetry when reviewing facial bone X-rays.

## McGrigor and Campbell's lines

These five lines can be used as an aid in the interpretation of facial bone X-rays (using both views). As well as use of the five lines, the symmetry of the face can also be used to help detect injury. If one side looks different from the other, there is a chance that this can be caused by trauma. Each line should run smoothly with no steps or breaks.

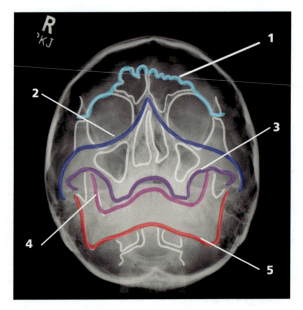

**Figure 6.5** X-ray showing the five lines of McGrigor and Campbell. © 2022 University Hospitals of North Midlands NHS Trust. All rights reserved.

### McGrigor's lines

**Line 1:** Runs from one zygomaticofrontal suture, across the forehead (assessing the frontal sinuses) and the supraorbital margin through to the opposite frontozygomatic suture. Assess for widening of the zygomaticofrontal suture, opacification or fluid levels within the frontal sinus, orbital emphysema ('black eyebrow' sign).

    **Line 2:** Passes along the superior aspect of the zygomatic arch and through the body of the zygoma, then passes through the infraorbital margin, over the bridge of the nose and then follows the same pattern across the opposite side of the face. Assess for superior zygomatic fractures, infraorbital fractures, soft-tissue opacity within the superior aspect of the maxillary sinus ('teardrop' sign). It is also important to check the nasal bones thoroughly to assess for fractures.

    **Line 3:** Runs along the inferior margin of the zygomatic arch, through the lateral and inferior walls of the maxillary sinus, across the maxilla (assessing the teeth) and following the same pattern across the opposite side of the face. Assess for inferior zygomatic fractures, fluid levels or opacification within the maxillary sinus and fractures of the alveolar ridge and upper teeth.

## Campbell's lines

**Line 4:** Runs from the mandibular ramus and through the superior aspect of the mandible to the opposite ramus. Assess for fractures of the superior aspect of the mandible and assess the lower teeth.

**Line 5:** Travels from the mandibular condyle through the inferior aspect of the mandible to the opposite condyle. Assess for fractures of the inferior aspect of the mandible, assess the angle of mandible and body as these regions are susceptible to fracture.

## Soft-tissue signs of facial trauma

The soft-tissue signs indicating facial trauma can be subtle at times so careful and thorough examination is required.

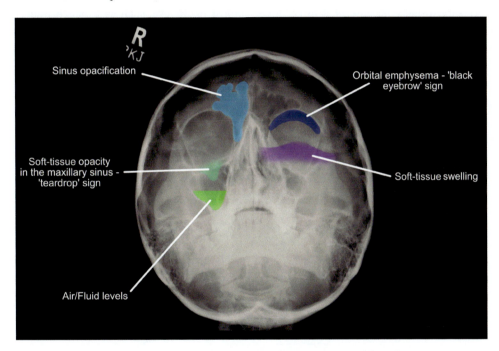

**Figure 6.6** X-ray demonstrating the common soft-tissue signs of facial trauma. © 2022 University Hospitals of North Midlands NHS Trust. All rights reserved.

**Sinus opacification:** Opacification of the sinus may be due to acute trauma (blood-filled ethmoid or maxillary sinus) or other conditions (sinusitis).

**'Black Eyebrow' sign:** The black eyebrow sign is a curvilinear region of air that collects in the superior aspect of the orbit and is usually associated with an orbital fracture. When the fracture occurs, air from the sinus (usually maxillary but can also originate from the ethmoid sinus) leaks into the orbital region and rises to the superior aspect of the orbit, giving it the appearance of an eyebrow on imaging. Be aware of the mimics of the black eyebrow sign including fat surrounding the orbit or patients with sunken eyes; both of these can mimic the black eyebrow sign, however, they tend to be bilateral.

**Soft-tissue swelling:** Swelling is always a good indicator of injury, and it is important to carefully assess the regions with swelling. However, it does not always indicate a fracture and may just demonstrate soft-tissue injury.

**Air/Fluid levels:** Typically seen in the maxillary sinus and is a sign of fluid (usually blood) build-up within an air-filled structure. The presence of an air/fluid level is usually an indicator of fracture, even if one cannot be seen (occult). When in the maxillary sinus, the presence of fluid usually indicates a fracture in the orbital floor. If the imaging is performed with the patient supine, the fluid will pool at the posterior aspect of the sinus and will cause a generalised opaque appearance, which can easily be mistaken for chronic pathologies. For this reason, erect facial bone X-rays are preferred.

'Teardrop' sign: The teardrop sign is a soft-tissue opacity that develops at the superior aspect of the maxillary sinus and is caused by herniation of orbital content such as fat through the orbital floor, usually as a result of trauma to the eye. Increased intra-orbital pressure (usually because of a direct force applied to the eye, such as a punch injury), causes a fracture to the orbital floor, which is a very thin layer of bone. Fat and muscle herniate through the fracture into the superior aspect of the maxillary sinus, creating a teardrop-like opacity on imaging. This appearance is associated with an orbital blow out fracture. In paediatric patients, the fracture fragment may move back into place, entrapping the herniated tissue. In these cases, patients will present with diplopia (double vision) on upwards gaze, enophthalmos (sunken eye) and infraduction of the affected eye.

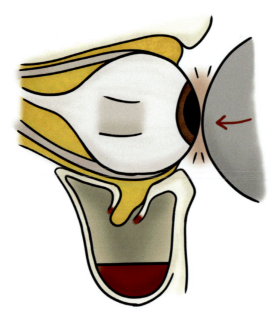

**Figure 6.7** An illustration demonstrating the mechanism involved with a orbital blow out fracture.

## Cartilage and joints of the face

The sutures seen within the face should be equal in size bilaterally. If there is widening present, it may indicate an acute injury in that region. However, always check to see if the image is rotated as rotation can lead to distortion of structures such as the sutures making them appear widened. The condylar processes should sit within the temporomandibular joints (TMJs). If assessing the TMJs, consider true mandible X-ray, including the lateral oblique views or an orthopantomogram (OPG).

## Fractures of the upper third of the face

Fractures in this region are unusual and include fractures of the frontal bone, extended nasoethmoid fracture and supraorbital region. Patients may present with epistaxis, soft-tissue swelling and deformity, cerebrospinal fluid rhinorrhoea, anaesthesia of the infraorbital nerve and pain on upwards gaze. When a fracture within the region is suspected, CT facial bone imaging is recommended.

## Tripod fractures (zygomaticomaxillary complex fractures)

Tripod fractures are associated with direct blow or injury to the cheek or zygomatic arch which results in a fracture involving the frontal process of the zygoma, the zygomatic arch and the superior and lateral wall of the maxillary sinus. Clinical findings can include soft-tissue swelling and facial distortion with the cheek bones appearing lower on the affected side. On X-ray imaging, fracture fragments may be difficult to see if there is no significant displacement so it is vital to check for the other radiological signs of fracture, such as an air/fluid level.

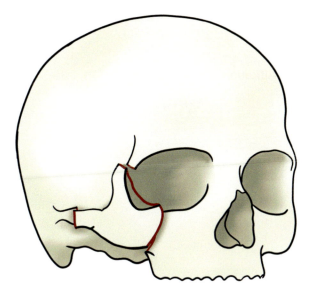

**Figure 6.8** A tripod fracture.

## Le Fort classifications

Le Fort fractures are fractures that involve the midface which fall into three categories.

- **Le Fort 1:** A fracture of the maxilla resulting in separation of the teeth from the rest of the skull. Results from a fracture of the medial and lateral walls of the maxillary sinus and the nasal septum.
- **Le Fort 2:** A triangular-shaped fracture extending from the maxilla towards the nasofrontal suture. The fracture lines run inferiorly and laterally through the medial and inferior walls of the orbit, through the lateral walls of the maxillary sinus with a fracture of the nasal septum (which can be at variable levels).
- **Le Fort 3:** A transverse fracture extending through the nasal bones at the superior aspect, through the medial and lateral walls of the orbits and extending into the zygomatic arches or sutures.

These fractures tend to result from a direct blow to the midface, usually seen in RTCs or alleged assaults. X-ray will not fully demonstrate the severity of the fracture and may underestimate the severity of the maxillary and orbital fractures; in these cases, CT facial bones is preferred.

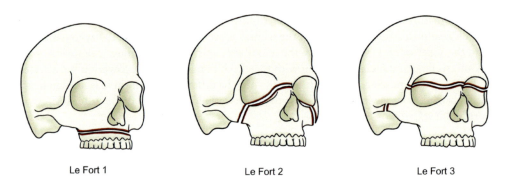

Le Fort 1  Le Fort 2  Le Fort 3

**Figure 6.9** Le Fort classification of facial fractures.

# Mandible

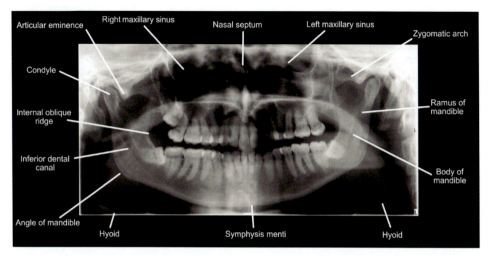

**Figure 6.10** An orthopantomogram (OPG) showing the anatomy of the mandible.

## Fractures of the mandible

The mandible is considered a ring-bone structure, so it is common for fractures to occur in more than one place. Therefore, if one fracture is identified always check for a secondary one. Mandible injury is commonly a result of moderate energy transfer to the lower face, frequently seen in alleged assaults, falls and RTAs. Patients present with alteration in their bite, pain, swelling, paraesthesia or anaesthesia to the alveolar nerve, inability to open mouth, bleeding from the ear and sublingual haematoma.

Fractures tend to occur at a point of weakness along the mandible or due to other underlying bony pathology.

- The mandibular condyle is an anatomically thin region of bone.
- The angle of the mandible is a weakness, especially when there is an un-erupted third molar present.
- The paraphyseal region is weak due to the long root of the canines.
- The body of the mandible is prone to injury from trauma, such as direct blow.
- The symphysis is prone to injury following a fall with direct blow to the chin.
- Injury to the condyles and TMJs can be difficult to identify (especially on lateral oblique mandible X-rays).

In paediatric patients, the incomplete dentition can help add strength to the mandible and help prevent fracture. Fractures of the condylar and sub-condylar regions are more common in paediatric patients.

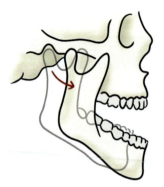

## Temporomandibular joint dislocation

The most common type of TMJ dislocation is an anterior dislocation. Posterior, superior and lateral dislocations are less commonly seen. It tends to occur from excessive opening of the mouth. The mandibular condyle is abnormally displaced, causing a loss of normal articulation which can lead to the mouth being stuck open. Patients present with pain at the TMJ, with an inability to close the mouth with difficulty speaking, protrusion of the chin and excessive salivation.

**Figure 6.11** TMJ dislocation.

## Dentition

Adults have 32 permanent and children have 20 deciduous teeth. Individual adult teeth can be identified using a system that divides the mouth into quadrants with numbers 1 to 8 used to identify each tooth, starting with the central incisor at number 1 to the third molar at number 8. Deciduous teeth are identified slightly differently. The mouth is still divided into quadrants, however, the letters A to E are used to identify the five teeth in each quadrant. The central incisor is identified as A extending to the molars which are identified as E.

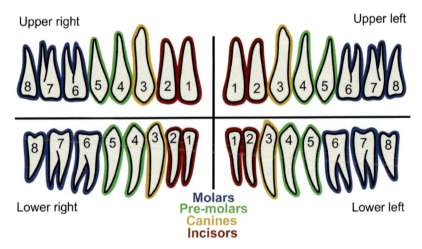
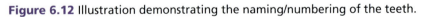

**Figure 6.12** Illustration demonstrating the naming/numbering of the teeth.

Each tooth is comprised of a central pulp (which contains all the neurovascular structures) surrounded by a dense outer layer of cementum. This continues up to the crown where this layer thickens to form enamel. Teeth sit within a bony socket lined by the lamina dura with the periodontal ligament responsible for holding the tooth in place.

Teeth can be injured following trauma or can sustain damage from more chronic conditions. Commonly seen pathologies include:

- **Periapical lucencies:** Widening or loss of the continuity with the lamina dura usually indicating periapical disease. Patients present with acute history of pain with a lucency seen on imaging surrounding the root.
- **Caries:** Demineralisation of the tooth's surface usually associated with bacterial infection.

OPG imaging is good at demonstrating the condition of the dentition, which cannot always be visualised on mandible X-rays.

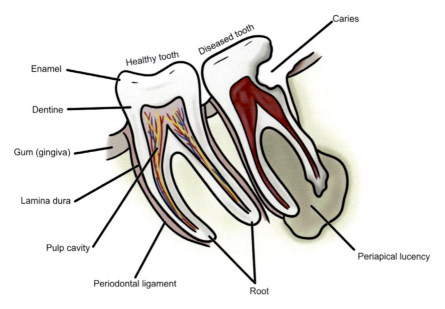

**Figure 6.13** Illustration demonstrating a healthy tooth and its anatomy and a diseased tooth.

## Paediatric skull and face

Bony facial injury in infants (under 5s) is rare and X-rays of paediatric facial bones are contra-indicated in patients under 5 years as the patient is likely to have suffered further head injury and CT imaging is indicated in these cases and is recommended by the NICE guidelines. As the age of the patient progresses, so does the incidence of injury to the facial region. The structure of the paediatric skull and face means that the forehead will take the brunt of the trauma within this region.

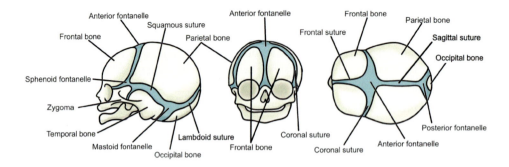

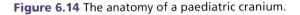

**Figure 6.14** The anatomy of a paediatric cranium.

## Sutures and fontanelles

There are six major fontanelles found at the four corners of the parietal bones; accessory fontanelles can be found within the sagittal suture. The posterior fontanelle may be closed at birth, but usually closes within 2 months pre-natal to 2 months post-natal. The anterior fontanelle closes by 12–18 months.

In the post-natal period, the sutures may appear wider than normal due to membranous ossification being incomplete but will close 'clinically' at 6–12 months. The coronal, lambdoid and sagittal sutures will persist throughout childhood (and generally do not fully ossify until the age of 30).

## Patterns of injury

Falls are the most common mechanism seen within patients under 5 and are usually not complicated by intracranial injury. As the patient ages RTCs become the most commonly seen mechanism of injury (5–13-year-olds). These are usually associated with high-energy trauma. Pedestrian RTC is the most common cause of death from head injury.

Be aware of non-accidental injury (NAI) especially in a patient under the age of 5 with multiple physical injuries to the head and neck, missing or broken teeth and multiple fractures of different ages with malunion or nonunion. Changing or inconsistent mechanisms of injury should also raise the suspicion of NAI.

## Signs of injury

- Soft-tissue swelling
- Steps or widening in the sutures – sutures should have a sclerotic border within typical positions and should be easily identifiable from a fracture
- Cortical breaks
- Densities within the cranium, which can indicate a depressed fracture.

# Systematic Assessment – Facial Bones

## AABCS

- Anatomy and image quality
- Alignment
- Bones
- Cartilage
- Soft tissues

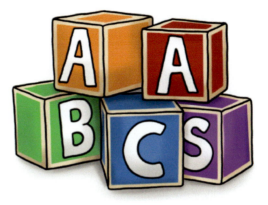

**Figure 6.15** AABCS building blocks.

## Anatomy and image quality

Ensure the images are for the correct patient and are the most recent and up-to-date images. Is all the required anatomy demonstrated? Are the images of a good diagnostic quality? If not, consider why the images are of poor quality. It may be due to the technique used by the radiographer such as the exposures used or the patient positioning, it may be due to factors beyond the control of the radiographer such as patient body habitus or condition. External artefacts such as clothing, immobilisation aids or splints can mask anatomy or pathology.

## Alignment

Check the five lines of McGrigor and Campbell. These should be smooth with no steps or jumps within the lines. Check that the facial bones are symmetrical when compared to the opposite side. Lack of symmetry can indicate acute injury.

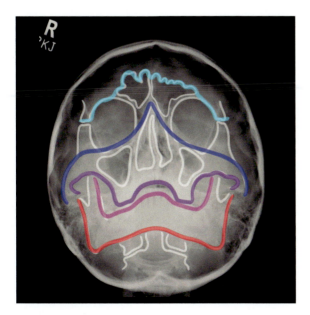

**Figure 6.16** X-ray showing the five lines of McGrigor and Campbell. © 2022 University Hospitals of North Midlands NHS Trust. All rights reserved.

## Bones

Check each cortex individually – steps, breaks or acute angles in the cortical outline can indicate acute injury. Check the medulla, assessing for lucency.

Don't forget to assess the mandible!

## Cartilage

Check the sutures are preserved with no widening or crowding of the joint spaces. Re-assess the joint alignment, including assessment of the mandible.

## Soft tissues

Check for soft-tissue swelling. This can usually be assessed better on the OM30 projection, especially if the swelling involves the infraorbital region.

Assess for facial symmetry.

Check for fluid levels or opacities within the sinus. Is there a 'teardrop' sign? Is there a 'black eyebrow' sign?

# Chapter 7

# Paediatric Skeleton

## Overview

This chapter begins with an introduction to the anatomy of the epiphysis and an explanation of the different injuries that can occur in growing bone.

Following on from this will be an overview of common paediatric trauma in different body regions, finally there will be an introduction to non-accidental injury in infants and children and the common presentations and warning signs.

## Anatomy of the Epiphyseal Plate

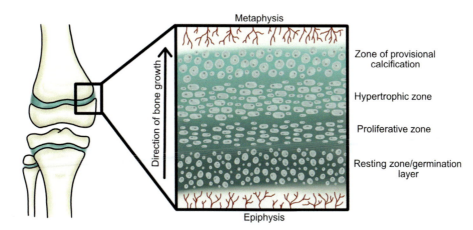

**Figure 7.1** Anatomy of the epiphyseal plate.

The role of the epiphyseal plate or physis is longitudinal bone growth in the immature skeleton. Cartilage is produced and then remodelled into bone cells. Within the physis are several different layers, each with different functions in the growth of bone.

**Germination layer:** Also known as the resting zone. This is the layer closest to the epiphysis and where chondrocytes (cartilage cells) are produced. These cells are essential for bone growth and any injury to this zone can result in growth cessation.

**Proliferation zone:** This is where the chondrocytes divide, flatten, and begin to organise into columns. This is what causes the epiphysis to grow. Any injury to this zone can result in growth cessation.

**Hypertrophic zone:** The chondrocyte columns lengthen; the cells then mature and die. There is no active growth in this region, and it is the weakest part of the physis. Because of this weakness, it is a common site of injury.

**Zone of provisional calcification:** This is where the chondrocytes calcify and become osteoblasts and then through the process of maturity develop into osteophytes. If there is any injury at this region, the bone will heal normally.

## Salter-Harris classifications

In the paediatric skeleton, there is the possibility of injury to the epiphyseal plate following trauma that results in a fracture in the region of the epiphysis. The most common sites for fractures involving the epiphysis are the distal radius, distal humerus and the ankle.

The Salter-Harris classification system uses five grades to describe the fracture pattern, the higher the grading scale, the more severe the fracture. When classifying Salter-Harris, orientate the image with the affected growth plate at the bottom. In the case of distal radius fracture, etc., this may involve turning the image to correctly classify the fracture.

The word **SALTER** can be used a mnemonic for the Salter-Harris classification system:

S   – Slipped – SH I
A   – Above (the growth plate) – SH II
L   – Lower (than the growth plate) – SH III
TE – Through Everything – SH IV
R   – Rammed (growth plate rammed into metaphysis) – SH V.

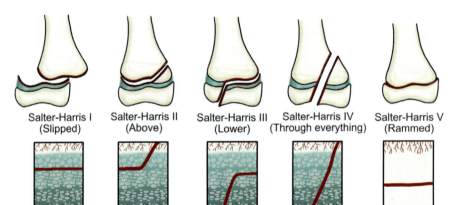

Salter-Harris I (Slipped) | Salter-Harris II (Above) | Salter-Harris III (Lower) | Salter-Harris IV (Through everything) | Salter-Harris V (Rammed)

**Figure 7.2** Different types of Salter-Harris fractures and the effect of the fracture on the microscopic anatomy of the epiphyseal plate.

## Salter-Harris I (Slipped)

A fracture of the physis only, resulting in the epiphysis slipping out of alignment with the metaphysis. The fracture line passes through the hypertrophic zone and zone of provisional calcification and doesn't involve the growth zone. Growth disruption following this fracture is uncommon. A slipped upper femoral epiphysis (SUFE) is an example of an SH I.

## Salter-Harris II (Above)

A fracture through the physis which extends into the metaphysis. SH II fractures are the most commonly seen Salter-Harris fractures. The fracture doesn't involve the active growth zones of the epiphysis, and growth disruption following this type of fracture is rare.

## Salter-Harris III (Lower)

A fracture through the physis which extends into the epiphysis. This fracture line extends through the proliferating zone and involves a region of active growth as a result of this type of fracture. Growth disturbance may occur.

## Salter-Harris IV (Through Everything)

The fracture extends from the articular surface, through all layers of the physis and into the metaphysis. As the fracture involves all layers within the physis, there is a high risk of growth disturbance.

## Salter-Harris V (Rammed)

A crushing or compression type fracture involving the physis. SH V types are very rare and usually subtle on X-ray and there may be no obvious fracture line or angulation, which can lead to misdiagnosis. They have a very high complication rate and carry a risk of partial closure of the physis, which can result in major growth disturbance or deformity.

## Common Paediatric Trauma

### Elbow trauma

Supracondylar fractures are the most common type of paediatric elbow fractures. Most commonly seen in younger children from 3 to 10 years of age and typically results from a fall onto an outstretched hand (FOOSH) and extension type mechanisms. Patients will present with pain and reduced range of movement along with swelling and deformity if the fracture is displaced.

Lateral epicondyle fractures are the second most commonly seen elbow fracture. They are intra-articular fractures and it is important to recognise lateral condyle fractures and not mistake them for supracondylar fractures, as treatment, in the form of an open reduction and internal fixation (ORIF), is usually indicated.

Medial epicondyle fractures are less common and have a high association with dislocation, so assessment of elbow alignment is crucial when this type of fracture is suspected.

The ossification centres of paediatric patients are vulnerable to particular injuries. Each ossification centre begins to develop at different ages. Use CRITOL to assess development of the paediatric elbow.

CRITOL lists the sequence in which the ossification centres appear on X-ray:

1 Capitulum (1 year)
2 Radial head (3 years)
3 Internal (medial) epicondyle (5 years)
4 Trochlea (7 years)
5 Olecranon (9 years)
6 Lateral epicondyle (11 years).

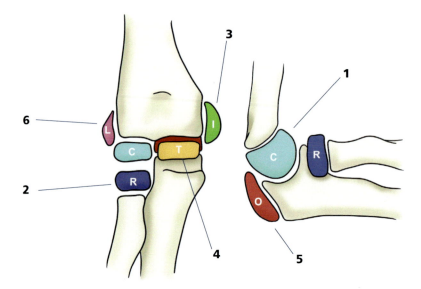

**Figure 7.3** Ossification centres of the elbow joint.

## Wrist and forearm trauma

Buckle fractures (also known as torus fractures) are very common in children aged 2–12 years. These fractures occur when one cortex is compressed (causing cortical bulging) and the opposite cortex remains intact. Commonly caused by axial loading through the bone, such as FOOSH when seen in the wrist. Patients will usually present with pain and swelling to the affected limb. X-ray images will demonstrate cortical bulging, however, in some cases, there may only be very subtle cortical angulation present.

The forearm is a common site for bowing deformity fractures. These occur primarily in children as the bones are soft in the immature skeleton and will bend rather than break when force is applied. As the force applied increases, a greenstick fracture may occur; this is when one cortex breaks and the other cortex remains intact.

## Knee trauma

Tibial eminence fractures are often seen at the insertion point of the anterior cruciate ligament (ACL). Avulsion fractures are seen as the tibial eminence is weak in comparison to the ligament in the immature skeleton. Commonly seen as a result of rotation and hyper-extension of the knee joint, usually as a result of sporting injury (such as sudden deceleration) or from a fall onto a hyper-extended leg. Patients will present with significant pain, inability to weight bear, reduced range of movement and swelling (usually with presence of a knee joint effusion). X-rays usually demonstrate a small bony fragment within the intracondylar notch, with the presence of associated effusion/lipohaemarthrosis.

Chondral/osteochondral lesions are common in children. Dependent upon what stage of skeletal maturity the child has reached, the location of the lesion can be different. In children with an open physis, femoral lesions are more common and, in children with a closed physis, lesions within the patella are more commonly seen. Patients present with pain, which is worse on activity, swelling and effusion and stiffness.

Osgood-Schlatters disease is a chronic avulsion and fragmentation of the tibial tuberosity. This can cause inflammation, patella tendon thickening and reactive bone formation. Patients will present with anterior knee pain, with swelling and tenderness over the tibial tuberosity. X-rays will demonstrate focal soft-tissue swelling over the tibial tuberosity and loss of definition of the patella tendon followed by fragmentation and irregularity of the tibial tuberosity.

Sinding-Larsen-Johnsson syndrome is similar to Osgood-Schlatter's but affects the patella tendon at the insertion point at the inferior aspect of the patella causing fragmentation of the inferior aspect of the patella with swelling and tendon thickening. Patients will present with anterior knee pain (localised to the inferior aspect of the patella) and focal soft-tissue swelling.

The patella sleeve fracture is unique to the paediatric population and is an avulsion fracture of the patella cartilage, commonly seen in 8–12-year-olds. These are seen as a result of contraction of the quadriceps and result in a small avulsion type fracture at the inferior aspect of the patella, with associated swelling, effusion and patella alta. Patients will present with localised pain at the inferior pole of the patella, soft-tissue swelling or effusion, reduced range of movement and a palpable high riding patella.

## Tibia and fibula

Toddler's fractures are a commonly seen spiral or oblique fracture of the tibial diaphysis, which is usually subtle and un-displaced and may only be visible on one of the X-ray views. These can occur from a minor injury such as twisting (due to the abnormal gait of a toddler) or falling. However, sometimes a parent may be unable to recall a trauma with the child presenting with refusal to weight bear, pain and swelling. These fractures are only seen in ambulatory patients. If seen in a very young infant or non-ambulatory patients, then a non-accidental injury (NAI) must be considered.

## Ankle

Tillaux fractures are a type of Salter-Harris II fracture typically seen in older children as the physis begins to fuse. The physis fuses from the medial aspect to the lateral aspect making the lateral aspect more susceptible to avulsion type injury in this age group. There is an external rotation/supination mechanism which results in an SH II avulsion fracture at the insertion point of the anterior tibiofibular ligament, and at the anterolateral aspect of the tibial epiphysis. Patients will present with pain, an inability to weight bear and swelling. However, significant deformity isn't usually seen as the fibula will normally prevent any significant fracture displacement.

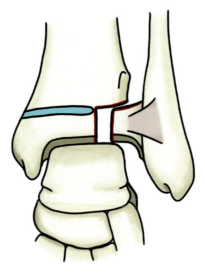

**Figure 7.4** Tillaux fracture.

Triplane fractures are a type of Salter-Harris IV fracture seen in adolescents and are made up of multiple fracture lines, usually seen as the result of external rotation/supination mechanisms (similar to Tillaux fractures). Fractures will occur in all three anatomical planes and usually comprise of a vertical fracture of the epiphysis, horizontal fracture of the physis and an oblique fracture of the metaphysis. Patients will present with pain and swelling, inability to weight bear and deformity of the ankle.

# Hip trauma

Developmental dysplasia of the hip (DDH) is an instability of the hip with associated subluxation or dislocation. X-ray is the best modality to assess after the age of 6 months. Prior to this, ultrasound is preferred as the femoral epiphysis doesn't begin to ossify until approximately 6 months of age.

AP X-rays can be used to assess the symmetry of the pelvis, acetabular angle, Shenton's line and the position and condition (density, size and location) of the femoral epiphysis.

- Shenton's lines should be smooth and the same on both sides (unless bilateral DDH) if there is disruption consider DDH.
- Hilgenreiner's line is a horizontal line running through the triradiate cartilage of both acetabula and can be used as a reference point for the position of Perkin's line, which is drawn perpendicular to Hilgenreiner's line and should intersect the lateral aspect of the acetabulum. In a normal paediatric pelvis, the femoral epiphysis should sit in the inferomedial aspect of the grid created by these two lines. If the femoral head is sitting laterally, DDH should be considered.
- The acetabular roof may be steeper in DDH (normal angle is 30°).

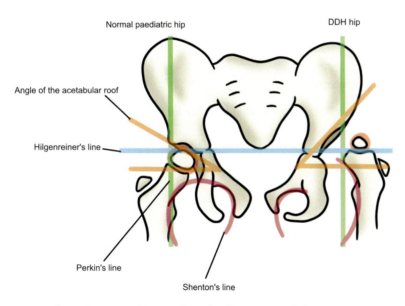

**Figure 7.5** The assessment lines and angles for DDH and their appearance on a normal pelvis (left) and a pelvis with DDH (right).

Perthes (Legg-Calve-Perthes) is osteonecrosis of the femoral epiphysis, not caused by trauma, and the changes differ from avascular necrosis caused by fracture or dislocation. Patients are usually aged between 4 and 10 years and present with atraumatic pain (coincidental history of trauma may be present) or limp. Blood tests usually come back normal. X-ray features of Perthes include joint effusions, subluxation, increased sclerosis and flattening of the femoral head. The condition is self-limiting and, over time, healing and remodelling of the femoral head will result in a normal appearance.

A SUFE is a Salter-Harris type I fracture involving the proximal femoral epiphysis. Seen more commonly in males between the ages of 10 and 17 years, this presents earlier in females (8–15 years). Obesity is considered a significant risk factor. Patients present with no history of trauma with a long-standing history of pain, limp, leg-length discrepancy or rotation and reduced range of motion.

AP and frog lateral X-rays are good for visualisation and will demonstrate widening of the femoral epiphysis and disruption of Klein's line. On the AP view, draw a line from the lateral aspect of the femoral neck (Klein's line). If this line **fails** to intersect the femoral epiphysis consider a SUFE. The frog lateral view demonstrates a SUFE better. The epiphysis usually slips posteriorly and medially.

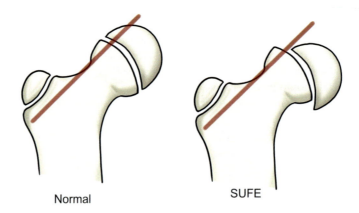

Normal                SUFE

**Figure 7.6** Normal appearance of a paediatric hip and a hip with a SUFE.

# Non-Accidental Injury/Suspected Physical Abuse

Accidental trauma is commonly seen in children and tends to occur in typical locations such as knees, elbows, tibia/fibula, forearm, chin, nose and forehead. Patients presenting to A&E with injuries in these regions, with appropriate mechanism of injury, should not normally raise the suspicion of physical abuse, unless frequency or other factors cause concern.

NAI tends to occur in specific locations with specific injury patterns seen. If the injury has occurred to an unusual location such as the eyes, cheeks, mouth, neck, upper arms, chest, back, buttocks, thighs and genitals with patients presenting with mechanisms of injury that would not normally cause injury to these regions, or with changing clinical history provided by parents/guardians/carers, then suspicion for NAI should be raised.

Other signs that can indicate NAI include untreated wounds or fractures, bruising that may reflect an imprint, bite marks, scalds, splash marks, tie marks, burns in unusual places, multiple burns, and bruising and injury to non-patients inconsistent with the patient's developmental age (such as a toddler's fracture in a non-ambulatory patient).

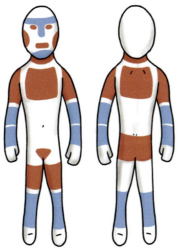

**Figure 7.7** Patterns of common accidental trauma in children – shown in blue, and patterns which should raise concern for NAI – shown in red.

Typical features associated with NAI:

- Obvious midshaft fracture
- Subtle injuries that may by indicated with subtle periosteal reaction
- Splaying of the metaphysis
- Corner/Bucket handle metaphyseal fractures
- Spiral (toddler's) fractures in non-ambulatory patients without a history of twisting commonly seen in the tibia and femur. A twisting-type injury should not be seen in non-ambulatory patients and a spiral fracture in this region can indicate a twisting force being applied to the limb from an external source. Spiral fractures may be seen in toddlers due to the abnormal twisting style gait seen in those learning to walk.

> ## TIP
>
> The most common site for NAI is the ribs, followed by the lower limbs and then the upper limb.

## Rib fractures

Rib fractures are a common sign of NAI and tend to affect multiple ribs. Non-displaced rib fractures are usually difficult to identify on X-ray. However, when the healing process begins, the fracture may become more obvious. Fractures of the neck/shaft of the rib are seen as widening of the fracture line followed by callus formation (visible 7–10 days post injury). Fractures at the head of the rib, however, may remain undetectable. Fractures of the posterior ribs are highly specific for inflicted injury.

Rib fractures in infants are an indicator of high-force injury. Due to the nature of the immature skeleton, lower force injury will not result in a fracture (as the bones are softer and more likely to bend). Rib fractures can be associated with other mechanisms such as birth trauma or premature birth and may be caused by metabolic disorders or bone dysplasia.

## Limb injury

When assessing limb injury in suspected NAI consider the type of fracture; transverse fracture of long bones usually implies a direct force has been applied. Oblique or spiral fractures in long bones tend to indicate a twisting type mechanism. In these cases, consider the age of the patient. Spiral fracture of the tibia is commonly seen in toddlers and an ambulatory patient so should not normally raise the suspicion of NAI. If these types of fractures have occurred in a non-ambulatory patient, such as an infant, then suspicion is higher. Location of the fracture can also indicate NAI. Fractures of the metaphyseal region are highly suspicious of NAI; corner fractures are subtle fractures that occur at the corner of the bone with a subcortical lucency seen, periosteal reaction can occur at the medial, lateral and distal aspect of the bone equalling a bucket handle appearance.

## Periosteal reaction

Periosteal reaction may not always be as a result of trauma. It may be an incidental finding related to an unexpected pathology, e.g. leukaemia, bone lesions, etc. In children under the age of 6 months, subperiosteal bone formation may be seen. This is a common finding in the developing bone and is usually seen in the tibia or femur. The appearance tends to be bilateral, less than 2 mm thick and will not extend past the metaphysis.

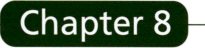

# Chapter 8

# Chest and Abdomen

## Overview

This chapter is a basic introduction to the complex regions of the thorax and the abdomen. An overview of basic thoracic trauma including fractures, pneumothoraces and effusion will be followed by an introduction to abdominal pathologies.

## Anatomy

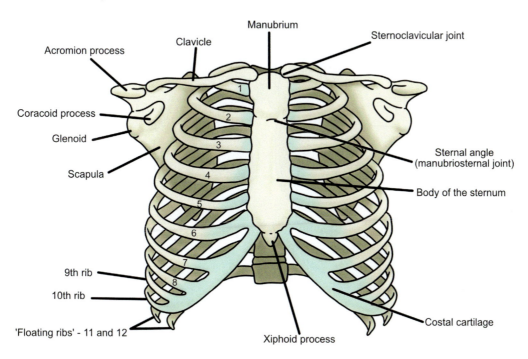

**Figure 8.1** Bony anatomy of the chest.

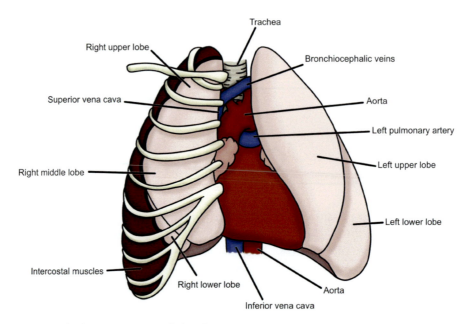

Trachea

Right upper lobe

Bronchiocephalic veins

Superior vena cava

Aorta

Left pulmonary artery

Left upper lobe

Right middle lobe

Left lower lobe

Intercostal muscles

Right lower lobe

Aorta

Inferior vena cava

**Figure 8.2** Soft-tissue anatomy of the chest.

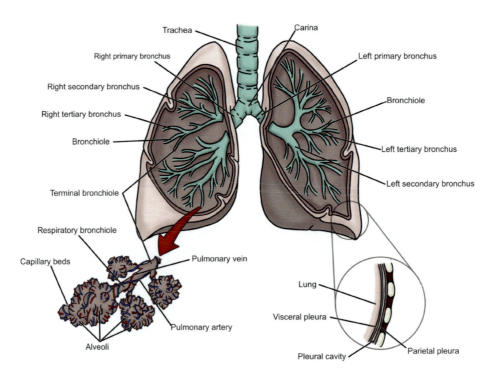

Trachea

Carina

Right primary bronchus

Left primary bronchus

Right secondary bronchus

Bronchiole

Right tertiary bronchus

Bronchiole

Left tertiary bronchus

Left secondary bronchus

Terminal bronchiole

Respiratory bronchiole

Capillary beds

Pulmonary vein

Lung

Visceral pleura

Pulmonary artery

Alveoli

Pleural cavity

Parietal pleura

**Figure 8.3** Anatomy of the lungs.

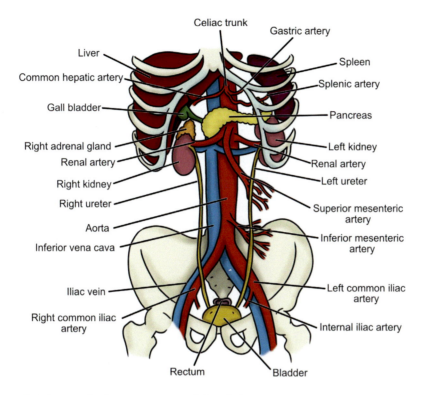

**Figure 8.4** Deep soft-tissue anatomy of the abdomen.

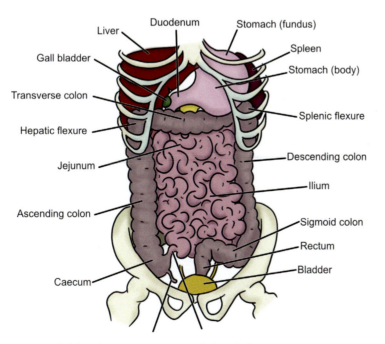

**Figure 8.5** Superficial soft-tissue anatomy of the abdomen.

# Chest Pathology – An Introduction

## Rib fractures

Rib fractures are a common consequence of trauma involving the chest. Chest X-rays are not indicated if a single or un-displaced fracture is suspected. These un-displaced fractures are often difficult to visualise on chest X-rays. However, if there are suspected complications, a chest X-ray can be indicated.

In cases involving chest trauma complications can include pneumothorax, haemathorax, pulmonary laceration and lung herniation, etc.

Fractures of the 4th to the 10th ribs are the most common. Fracture of the upper ribs (1st to 3rd) usually results from high-energy trauma and are associated with injury to the brachial plexus or the subclavian vascular region. Fractures of the lower ribs (10th to 12th) are associated with liver, renal and splenic injuries.

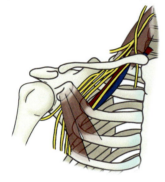

**Figure 8.6** The brachial plexus and the subclavian vascular region in relation to the upper ribs.

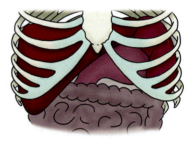

**Figure 8.7** The abdominal anatomy in relation to the lower ribs.

## Flail chest

A flail chest is defined as fractures of three or more continuous ribs in two or more places along the rib. This type of rib fracture is associated with high-energy trauma such as severe anteroposterior compression (such as in RTCs, crush type injury and blast forces). Clinically, the patient presents with a chest wall deformity, crepitus and paradoxical respiration.

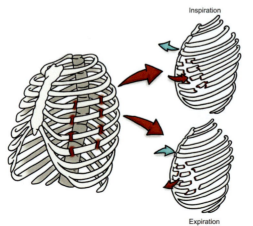

Inspiration

Expiration

**Figure 8.8** Illustration demonstrating paradoxical respiration.

**Paradoxical respiration:** The fractured section of the ribs (the flail segment) depresses into the chest with inspiration and expands with exhalation. This is the opposite to the normal chest breathing movement.

> **TIP**
>
> This can be a subtle finding at times, so thorough examination is required.

## Pneumothorax

Pneumothoraces occur when gas/air enters the pleural cavity causing the lung to collapse. There are three main ways air can enter the pleural cavity:

1. Perforation of the visceral pleura.
2. Perforation of the chest wall.
3. Gas formation due to microorganisms within the pleural cavity – however this is rare.

There are different ways of classifying a pneumothorax.

● According to how the air entered the pleural space:

 – **Closed pneumothorax:** Air within the pleural space without a penetrating wound through the chest wall but with rupture of the lung.
 – **Open pneumothorax:** Air enters through an opening or wound in the chest wall.
 – **Tension pneumothorax:** Air enters through an opening in the chest wall but is unable to leave due to the wound/opening acting as a valve. Pressure within the pleural cavity increases, which leads to compression of the structures on the contralateral side, such as compression of the mediastinum/heart and the opposite lung. Considered a life-threatening medical emergency with urgent decompression required.

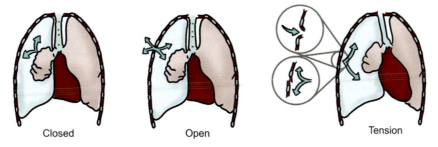

Closed          Open          Tension

**Figure 8.9** Illustration demonstrating the three types of pneumothorax according to how the air entered the pleural space – closed, open and tension.

> **TIP**
>
> Tension pneumothoraces should be considered a clinical, not a radiological diagnosis – if found should be treated first.

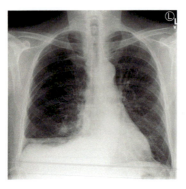

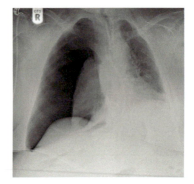

Figure 8.10 X-ray demonstrating a right apical pneumothorax. © 2022 University Hospitals of North Midlands NHS Trust. All rights reserved.

Figure 8.11 X-ray demonstrating a right pneumothorax demonstrating tension with mediastinal shift to the left. © 2022 University Hospitals of North Midlands NHS Trust. All rights reserved.

- According to how the pneumothorax occurs:

   - **Spontaneous pneumothorax:** Non-traumatic, a primary spontaneous pneumothorax happens when there are no underlying lung conditions. A secondary spontaneous pneumothorax results from underlying lung conditions.
   - **Traumatic pneumothorax:** Caused by invasive medical procedures such as line insertions, biopsy, etc. (iatrogenic) or following direct traumatic injury such as penetrating wounds, rib fractures, etc.

On X-ray, pneumothoraces appear as a thin white line at the lateral border of the lung. No lung markings can be seen past the pneumothorax (between the edge of the collapsed lung and the chest wall). If mediastinal shift is seen, a tension pneumothorax should be considered and the patient immediately reviewed.

## Haemothorax

This is a pleural effusion caused by blood within the pleural cavity, usually occurring from direct penetrating chest trauma. Patients present with shortness of breath with examination finding dull percussion, absent breath sounds and tachycardia/hypotension (possible shock symptoms due to blood loss). This can be seen on X-ray with blunting of the bases and if the haemothorax is large enough a meniscus will be seen. If the haemothorax occurs alongside a pneumothorax, these are called haemopneumothorax and can be seen on X-ray as an air/fluid line within the chest cavity with an associated pneumothorax.

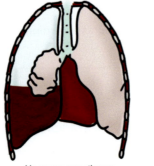

Haemopneumothorax

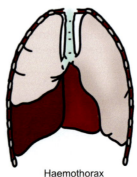

Haemothorax

Figure 8.12 Haemopneumothorax and haemothorax.

Both pneumothoraces and haemothoraces can be difficult to identify on supine chest X-rays as the air or fluid will gather at the anterior or posterior aspect of the chest cavity. In the case of a pneumothorax, the air will rise to the anterior aspect of the chest with the inflated lung behind giving the impression of normal lung unless a large pneumothorax develops. In the case of a haemothorax, the blood pools at the posterior aspect of the chest creating an opacification over the hemithorax.

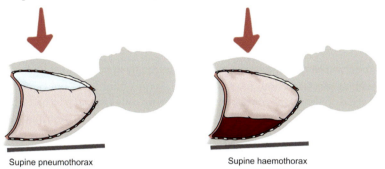

Supine pneumothorax          Supine haemothorax

**Figure 8.13** The effect of a supine patient position on a pneumothorax (air rising to anterior aspect of the chest cavity) and a haemothorax (blood pooling in posterior aspect of the chest cavity).

## Pleural effusion

A pleural effusion is a build-up of fluid within the pleural space. Normally, there is approximately 10–20 ml of fluid within the pleural space, which reduces friction between the parietal and visceral membrane layers when the patient breathes. The term pleural effusion can be used to describe any abnormal fluid collection within the pleura with limited specificity of the causes of the fluid build-up. The fluid can be caused by blood (haemothorax), serous fluid (hydrothorax) or pus (empyema/pyothorax).

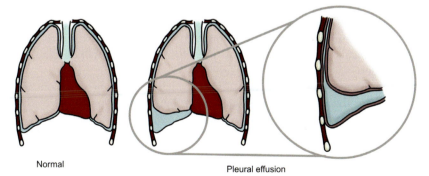

Normal                Pleural effusion

**Figure 8.14** Pleural effusion.

Small pleural effusions are difficult to identify on chest X-rays. There must be an accumulation of approximately 200–300 ml of fluid in the pleural space for it to be identified on an erect chest X-ray. The fluid collects in the lowest point of the chest cavity with blunting of the costophrenic angles being the first indicator of a pleural effusion. As the effusion increases in size, blunting of the cardiophrenic angle with the development of a homogenous opacification within the inferior aspect of the hemithorax will be seen.

Eventually, a 'meniscus sign' will develop as the pleural fluid develops higher at the lateral and medial border. In cases of large volume effusions, mediastinal shift and a reduction in lung volume may be present.

Supine chest X-rays are poor when trying to identify pleural effusions as the fluid pools in the posterior aspect of the chest and even large volume pleural effusions may be difficult to identify. Pleural effusions on supine chest X-rays can be seen as a hazy opacification overlying the whole hemithorax and can be misdiagnosed as consolidation or collapse.

## Consolidation

Consolidation within the lung occurs when the normally air-filled alveoli fill with a denser material such as pus (infection, i.e. pneumonia), serous fluid (pulmonary oedema), blood (haemorrhage or pulmonary contusion) or neoplastic cells (primary or metastatic cancer). Radiologically, each different material looks similar and clinical information should be used to help find a diagnosis.

X-ray features:

● Opacification within the lungs.
● **Air Bronchograms:** Air filled bronchus/bronchiole visible due to surrounding opacification.
● **Silhouette sign:** Helps determine which lobe the consolidation is in. In a normal chest X-ray, the outline of the mediastinum and diaphragm should be easily visible (the normal silhouette). When opacification is present, this normal outline/silhouette is lost. Different lobular consolidation affects the silhouette differently.

  – **Right upper lobe consolidation:** High up in the right lung, usually obscuring the normal silhouette. However, the right mediastinum contour may be lost.
  – **Right middle lobe consolidation:** Abuts the right atrium, thus consolidation will obscure the right heart border.
  – **Right lower lobe consolidation:** Abuts the right hemidiaphragm. Consolidation will obscure the right side of the diaphragm but does not usually affect the right heart border.
  – **Left upper lobe consolidation:** Consolidation will obscure the left aspect of the mediastinum and the left heart border.
  – **Left lingula consolidation:** Abuts the left ventricle and will obscure the left heart border.
  – **Left lower lobe consolidation:** Abuts the left hemidiaphragm. Consolidation will obscure the left side of the diaphragm, but usually do not affect the left heart border.
  – **Bilateral consolidation** can also be seen, e.g. 'batwing consolidation' which can be seen in a number of conditions such as pulmonary oedema, pneumonia, pulmonary haemorrhage, etc.

In some cases, it may be difficult to determine which lobe is affected by the consolidation, usually when the consolidation doesn't extend to the mediastinum. In these cases, it can be easier to describe the consolidation according to the 'zone' of which lung is being affected – upper, middle, or lower zone.

# Abdominal Pathology – An Introduction

Plain film imaging is best used as a preliminary investigation, with CT being better for further investigation and identification of suspected pathology.

Abdominal X-rays have limited value as they are restricted in what can be visualised (X-rays demonstrate gas, masses, bone and stones) so cannot fully exclude pathology. X-ray can be useful in the diagnosis of perforation, obstruction, and inflammatory bowel disease (mega colon, etc.). Visualisation of the small bowel on X-ray is limited as the small bowel is fluid filled.

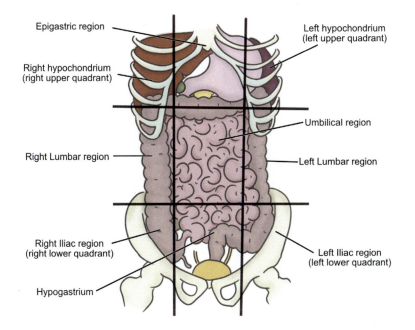

Epigastric region

Left hypochondrium
(left upper quadrant)

Right hypochondrium
(right upper quadrant)

Umbilical region

Right Lumbar region

Left Lumbar region

Right Iliac region
(right lower quadrant)

Left Iliac region
(left lower quadrant)

Hypogastrium

**Figure 8.15** Illustration demonstrating the abdominal regions.

## Small bowel obstruction

Small bowel obstruction (SBO) accounts for the majority of mechanical bowel obstructions. Commonly caused by adhesions (bands of scar-like tissues that develop between the abdominal organs), which are more commonly seen in developed countries or incarcerated hernias.

Patients present with cramps, acute pain, abdominal distension, nausea and vomiting. The radiographic appearance of an SBO includes dilated small bowel loops (measuring over 3.5 cm) with at least three or more loops visible. Dilated loops are usually seen in the central abdominal region. Small bowel can be identified as an acute/tight curvature with bowel folds (valvulae conniventes) usually visible.

## Large bowel obstruction

Large bowel obstructions (LBOs) are less common than SBOs. In adults, LBOs are commonly caused by colon cancer resulting in obstruction or acute diverticulitis. Patients present with pain, distension with associated nausea and vomiting with failure to pass stool/flatus.

Radiographic appearance includes distension or dilation of the bowel greater than 6 cm (or 9 cm in the caecum) with loss of the normal haustral folds.

### 3–6–9 rule

A guide to the normal measurements of the bowel. The small bowel should measure less than 3 cm, the large bowel and appendix should measure less than 6 cm and the caecum should measure less than 9 cm.

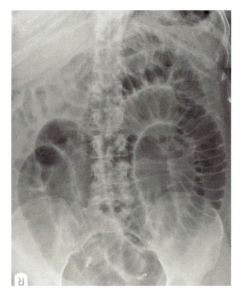

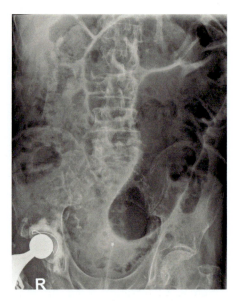

Figure 8.16 X-ray demonstrating an SBO. © 2022 University Hospitals of North Midlands NHS Trust. All rights reserved.

Figure 8.17 X-ray demonstrating an LBO. © 2022 University Hospitals of North Midlands NHS Trust. All rights reserved.

## Adynamic ileus

This is failure of passage of contents through the bowel (small or large); not a mechanical obstruction which represents paralysis of intestinal peristalsis. This can be symptomatic, but patients may also present with features of bowel obstruction, for example, abdominal distension, nausea and vomiting (bowel sounds may or may not be present).

This can be caused by several factors such as drug use, metabolic disorders, intra-abdominal inflammation, sepsis, congestive heart failure, myocardial infarction, head injury, abdominal trauma or surgery. Some degree of ileus is normal following abdominal surgery (including c-section), improving post-operative ileus can be determined clinically and radiologically.

Radiologically, the appearance includes uniform and gaseous bowel distension, which can be diffuse or localised (demonstrated with a sentinel loop).

## Intestinal volvulus

A broad term describing twisting of the bowel around its mesentery. Volvulus within the sigmoid region is the most common. Patients present with constipation, abdominal bloating and vomiting. Radiographically, this appears with large, dilated bowel loops with lack of haustra and rectal gas (coffee bean sign). Usually treated by a flatus tube, however, surgical intervention is occasionally required.

Caecal volvulus is rare but generally seen in younger patients. Patients present with pain, vomiting and abdominal distension. Radiographically, this appears with marked distension of the large bowel loops (caecal diameter greater than 9 cm) and a reduced haustral pattern.

## Pneumoperitoneum

This manifests as gas within the peritoneal cavity caused by a perforated viscus. There are multiple causes including peptic ulcer, ischaemic bowel, inflammatory bowel disease, obstruction and trauma. Post-operative free gas may be seen within the abdomen following abdominal surgery or laparotomy (always check for recent abdominal interventions).

Abdominal X-rays aren't sensitive for small volumes of free gas. However, erect chest X-rays may demonstrate small crescents of air below the hemidiaphragm. When large volumes of free gas are present, a double wall or 'Rigler's sign' will be seen as gas outlines both sides of the bowel.

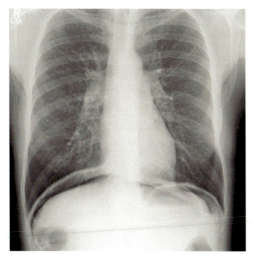

Figure 8.18 Erect chest X-ray demonstrating free air below the diaphragm suggesting a pneumoperitoneum. © 2022 University Hospitals of North Midlands NHS Trust. All rights reserved.

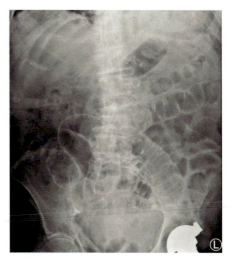

Figure 8.19 A supine abdominal X-ray demonstrating the Rigler's sign. © 2022 University Hospitals of North Midlands NHS Trust. All rights reserved.

## Inflammatory bowel disease (IBD)

**Ulcerative colitis:** Inflammatory disease of the colon. Typically affects younger patients (15–40 years). Patients present with pain, fever, and chronic diarrhoea. Inflammation begins at the anus and extends proximally. X-ray can demonstrate mural thickening, pneumatosis coli (intermural gas), thumb printing and a featureless descending colon with a block of faecal residue.

**Crohn's disease:** Idiopathic inflammatory bowel disease typically seen in patients between the ages of 15 and 25 years. Commonly affects the terminal ilium and proximal colon. Patients present with pain and chronic diarrhoea. X-ray demonstrates mural thickening, pneumatosis coli, thumb printing and a cobblestone appearance of the small and large bowel. MRI, CT and ultrasound are more accurate for assessment.

**Toxic megacolon:** A complication of IBD (commonly seen in infectious colitis): the colon (typically transverse) becomes dilated greater than 6 cm with loss of the haustral markings, pseudo polyps and sometimes thumb printing. Can sometimes cause perforation.

## TIPS

- Don't forget to assess the visualised lung bases (chest pathology can present with abdominal pain) – chest pathology can cause ileus, effusions can be secondary to abdominal pathology.
- Also check the visualised bones – check for fracture or pathology and consider dedicated imaging if needed

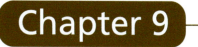

# Chapter 9

# Arthropathies

**Overview**

This chapter will introduce several commonly seen arthropathies, which includes degenerative diseases, erosive arthropathy and bone infection. We will cover the basic pathophysiology of the arthropathy as well as the different types of radiological appearances and distribution, followed by treatment options.

## Osteoporosis

Osteoporosis is a metabolic disease which involves a reduction in the bone mineral density causing a loss of bony trabecula and bone strength, typically as a result of reduced bone formation or an increase in bone reabsorption.

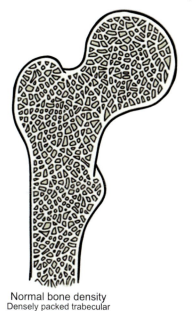 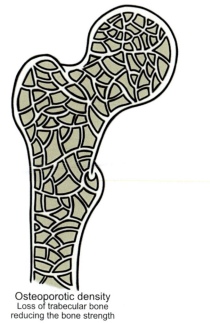

Normal bone density
Densely packed trabecular
bone adding strength

Osteoporotic density
Loss of trabecular bone
reducing the bone strength

**Figure 9.1** Differences between normal bone density and osteoporotic bone density.

Osteopenia can be classified into two broad categories – generalised osteopenia and localised osteopenia. Generalised osteopenia has several different causes, such as metabolic changes, deficiency with blood flow or congenital conditions. However, generalised osteopenia is often seen as a result of post-menopausal changes or progressing age (senile) which is classified as primary osteopenia.

Post-menopausal osteopenia (also known as Type 1 osteoporosis) typically occurs in older females and is related to reduced oestrogen levels following the menopause. This results in a loss of cancellous bones, followed later by a slower loss of cortical bone. Regions with high levels of cancellous bone are commonly affected, such as the hips, spine, and the metaphysis/epiphysis of long bones.

Age-related or senile osteopenia (also known as Type 2 osteoporosis) is caused by a reduction in the rate of bone formation, leading to a loss of both cortical and cancellous bone. Women are more commonly affected as men tend to develop more bone mass during puberty, thus the effects of reduced bone formation are less evident as they age.

Localised osteopenia is when there is a reduction in bone density in one specific region of the body. There are a number of different causes of localised osteopenia including infection, pain, disuse or immobilisation (e.g. following trauma and treatment with cast) or conditions such as complex regional pain syndrome or transient regional osteoporosis. This is classified as secondary osteopenia, which also accounts for osteopenia caused by endocrine diseases, such as diabetes, medication use and nutritional deficiency.

## Radiographic appearance

- **Altered trabecular pattern:** Trabecular loss tends to occur sequentially with the non-weight-bearing region losing structure first followed by the weight-bearing region (this can lead to the weight-bearing trabeculae appearing more prominent).
- Between 30–50% of bone loss is needed to be able to visualise it on plain film. Prominent sites to check are the proximal femur and hips. The Singh index can be used to assess the severity of osteoporosis. It uses a 6-tier grading system with normal healthy bone being categories as 'Grade 6' bone, with the bone decreasing in quality to the lowest, 'Grade 1'. Any bone categorised as 'Grade 3' or under is considered osteopenic.
- **Cortical thinning:** Normal bony cortex should account for one-third of the bone's width.

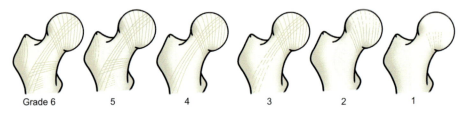

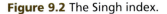
Grade 6      5      4      3      2      1

**Figure 9.2** The Singh index.

X-ray imaging is not considered sensitive enough to confirm an osteoporosis diagnosis. DEXA (dual energy X-ray absorptiometry) is considered the gold standard for diagnosis. DEXA scans use low energy X-rays to calculate the density of the bone according to how much of the delivered radiation is absorbed by the bone. If the bone has low density, then less radiation is absorbed, which may indicate osteoporosis.

Patients with osteoporosis and reduced bone density are more at risk of fractures as a result of low-energy trauma, due to the bones being weaker and more fragile. These types of fractures are classified as fragility fractures and will result from lower energy trauma, such as a fall from standing height, which in a patient with normal bone density would not result in a fracture.

Common sites for these types of injury include the wrist, pelvis and hip. Reduction in bone density also commonly affects the spine, which can lead to osteoporotic fractures – usually anterior wedge fractures.

## Osteoarthritis

Osteoarthritis (OA) is a degenerative joint disease and is the most commonly seen non-inflammatory arthropathy. It can affect any synovial joint but is typically seen in large weight-bearing joints, such as the hips and knees and in the axial skeleton. It is commonly seen in the active joints of the hands and feet, typically affecting the distal interphalangeal joints (DIPJs) and the proximal interphalangeal joints (PIPJs) and specifically the thumb carpometacarpal joint (CMCJ) and the metatarsophalangeal joint (MTPJ) of the great toe. OA can demonstrate a range of distributions affecting a single joint (monoarthritic) or multiple joints (polyarthritis) and is typically asymmetrical in distribution.

OA can be divided into primary or secondary OA. Primary OA refers to an idiopathic degenerative change, with no underlying conditions or direct cause and generally as a result of 'wear and tear' of the affected joint. Secondary OA refers to degenerative joint changes which are secondary to trauma (including joint surgery), inflammatory conditions such as rheumatoid arthritis (RA) or gout or increased force on the joint, such as obesity.

Patients typically present with joint pain and stiffness with joint instability. Symptoms are exacerbated by activity and may be relieved with rest.

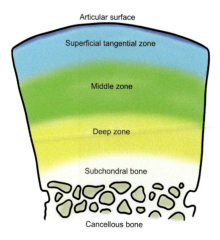

Understanding the anatomy and physiology of the articular surface is important in understanding the radiographic appearance of OA. The articular surface is made up of hyaline, which has a low coefficient to friction. It withstands compression, shearing and loading forces.

The articular surface is made up of several layers and is very poor at repairing itself. If the injury does not pass through all the layers, down to the subchondral bone it will not repair itself. In full depth injury to the articular surface, the cartilage will repair with fibrocartilage (not hyaline), which does not withstand forces such as compression as well as hyaline.

**Figure 9.3** Microscopic appearance of the articular surface.

## Radiographic appearance

X-rays are the first-line investigation for OA. The typically radiographic appearance of OA can be remembered with the mnemonic **LOSS**.

- **Loss of joint space:** This is caused by the thinning of the articular cartilage. In OA, the loss of joint space tends to be asymmetric and may be localised to one specific part of the joint. In specific joints such as the knee, weight-bearing X-rays can demonstrate the joint space narrowing more accurately than supine X-rays as the mechanical forces can demonstrate more severe narrowing and loss of joint alignment.
- **Osteophyte formation:** Bony lumps or spurs that develop at the periphery of the articular surfaces. These develop because of increased pressure on the joint and are the body's response to increased pressure by increasing the available surface area of the joint. Prominent osteophytes can cause restricted joint movement or impingement. Examples of this include osteophyte formation in the hands resulting in Heberden's nodes (affecting the DIPJs) or Bouchard's nodes (affecting the PIPJs). Prominent osteophyte formation at the MTPJ of the great toe can result in significantly reduced movement and is known as hallux rigidus.
- **Subchondral sclerosis:** Seen as an increase in bone density below the articular surface of the joint which can be caused by compression of the subchondral bone at the affected joint or by the body encouraging bone growth in the affected area as a response to the stress on that joint. As the disease progresses, the articular surface may begin to remodel.
- **Subchondral cyst:** Also known as geodes. These are seen as focal rounded peri-articular lucencies. In OA, subchondral cysts are usually caused by increased pressure within the joint forcing synovial fluid to herniate into the subchondral bone.

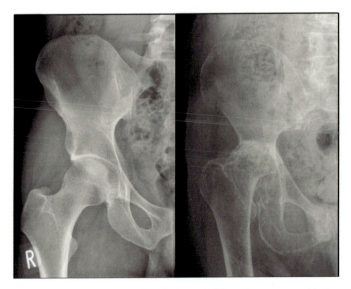

**Figure 9.4** X-rays showing a normal hip (on the left) with preserved joint spaces and no significant degeneration, and a hip demonstrating severe OA (on the right) with complete loss of the superior joint space, osteophyte and cystic formation, increased articular sclerosis and remodelling of the femoral articular surface. © 2022 University Hospitals of North Midlands NHS Trust. All rights reserved.

## Killgren-Lawrence classification system

This system is commonly used as a classification of OA severity. It can be used in the assessment and grading of OA affecting the hands (on the DP image), hips, knees, feet and c-spine (using the lateral image). The system uses 5 grades with 0 being considered normal ranging to the most severe – Grade 4.

- Grade 0 = Normal.
- Grade 1 = Early/minor. Doubtful joint space narrowing with possible osteophytosis.
- Grade 2 = Mild. Minimal joint space narrowing. Definite small osteophyte formation.
- Grade 3 = Moderate. Definite joint space narrowing with multiple moderately sized osteophytes. Subchondral sclerosis and possible deformity to the articular surface.
- Grade 4 = Severe. Marked joint space narrowing, multiple or large osteophytes, marked sclerosis and definite bony deformity.

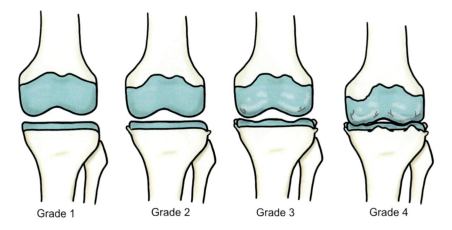

| Grade 1 | Grade 2 | Grade 3 | Grade 4 |

**Figure 9.5** The Killgren-Lawrence (Grade 1 – Grade 4) classification.

## Rheumatoid Arthritis

RA is the most common type of inflammatory arthritis and is a chronic autoimmune disease. It predominately affects the synovial tissues, however, it can also affect other organs and tissues such as the cardiovascular and pulmonary systems. It is a polyarthritis usually affecting the small joints of the hand, wrist and feet, including the metacarpophalangeal joints (MCPJs) and the PIPJs of the hands and the MTPJs and PIPJs of the feet.

Patients are typically middle aged and present with pain and morning stiffness of the affected joints. The affected joints may also swell, and blood tests will usually show positive Rheumatoid factor. Prompt diagnosis and referral is vital as rapid treatment improves the outcomes of RA and reduces the likelihood of significant joint damage. Treatment is aimed at relieving symptoms (pain and swelling) and slowing the disease progression. Treatment involves a combination of drugs such as non-steroidal anti-inflammatory drugs (NSAIDs) and drugs which suppress the immune system.

RA can also affect the paediatric population. Juvenile RA is a common chronic arthritic disease. Patients must present with symptoms under the age of 16 and those symptoms must last longer than 6 weeks. Patients present with pain which is worse in the morning but maintains throughout the day.

## Pathophysiology of rheumatoid arthritis

An antigen reaches the synovial tissues causing a local immune response, which causes synovitis (inflammation of the synovium). This leads to synovial hyperplasia (tissue enlargement) and formation of a pannus. The edge of the pannus contains cells that produce protease. this destroys the articular cartilage and osteoclasts are formed which destroy the subchondral bone causing erosions to occur.

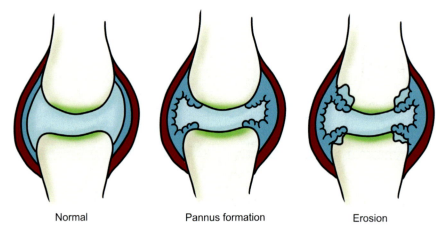

| Normal | Pannus formation | Erosion |

**Figure 9.6** Pathophysiology of RA, demonstrating the formation of the pannus and the resulting bony erosions.

## Radiographic appearance

- **Soft-tissue swelling:** Can be seen as a result of synovitis, joint effusions and the formation of the pannus. The effusions may cause the joint spaces to become slightly wider, however, this progresses to joint space narrowing as the cartilage erodes.
- **Osteopenia:** This is typically peri-articular and is a result of reduced bone density. This will become more pronounced as the disease progresses.
- Soft-tissue swelling and osteopenia are the first radiographic sign of RA.
- **Bony erosions:** Synovial inflammation invades and destroys the cartilage and the bone adjacent to the joint. The high protein levels within the synovial fluid can also cause this to happen. In RA, this is often referred to as 'marginal' or 'juxta-articular' erosions and is a classic appearance of RA.
- **Joint space narrowing:** The cartilage is damaged due to the persistent inflammation. Typically, the narrowing is symmetrical and uniform across the joint. This is best demonstrated in the hip joint. When the hip is affected by RA, it is common to see protrusion of the femoral head into the acetabulum, unlike in OA where superior migration due to the weight bearing forces, is more common.

As the disease progresses into the later stages, secondary signs such as remodelling of the joint subluxation/dislocations and deformity, due to the extensive erosion, can occur. Significant damage to the joint can result in secondary OA and the joint may also demonstrate osteophyte formation, subchondral sclerosis and subchondral cyst formation.

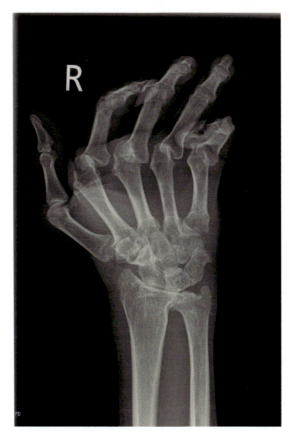

**Figure 9.7** X-ray demonstrating the classic signs of RA showing osteopenia, joint space narrowing, bone erosion and subluxations. © 2022 University Hospitals of North Midlands NHS Trust. All rights reserved.

# Psoriatic Arthritis

Psoriatic arthritis (PsA) is a chronic inflammatory arthritis usually developing alongside the skin condition psoriasis. There is a genetic link with the *HLA-B27* gene, so may be associated with other conditions including inflammatory bowel disease or eye disease.

PsA typically affects multiple joints with an asymmetrical distribution. It can affect a range of different joints but is commonly seen at the DIPJs of the fingers, the spine (including the SI joints) and large joints such as the hips and knees. The distribution of PsA can be described using the five main subtypes described below:

- Involving the DIPJs of the fingers and toes.
- Asymmetrical distribution affecting multiple joints (oligoarticular, affecting four or less joints). This distribution is usually seen at the knees and small joints.
- Symmetrical distribution affecting multiple joints, with a similar distribution to RA.
- Spondylarthritis, involving the spine and SI joints.
- Arthritis mutilans which is the most severe and destructive form of PsA with deformity of the fingers and toes seen.

Patients are typically middle aged and present with a history of psoriasis with pain, stiffness and swelling at the affected joints, usually in an asymmetrical pattern. Treatment of PsA often involves both rheumatology and dermatology input and depending on the severity of the symptoms, patients may require NSAIDs or disease-modifying anti-rheumatic drugs (DMARDs).

## Radiographic appearance

Radiographic appearance can depend on the area affected by PsA.

- **Soft tissue swelling:** Caused by joint, tendon and soft-tissue swelling and inflammation of an entire digit – finger or toe (dactylitis).
- **Bony changes:** Including erosions, which are usually well defined, these are similar to RA as they appear in a peri-articular location. However, unlike RA, the distribution of the erosions will be asymmetrical in distribution. Bony erosions may develop into 'pencil in cup' erosions, which is a severe form of erosions with destruction of the phalanx tip giving it a pointed appearance alongside new bone formation at the adjacent phalanx.
- New bone formation may be present giving a 'fluffy' appearance to the bones and is often seen alongside bone erosions. Further bone formation may be seen as enthesopathy at the attachment points of tendons and ligaments.
- **Periostitis:** Inflammation of the periosteum seen as an increased density adjacent to the cortex.

● **Spinal changes:** Sacroiliitis with irregular margins and sclerosis which can make visualisation of the SI joints difficult. This is caused by bony erosion and new bone formation. Spondylitis with bony proliferation throughout the spine.

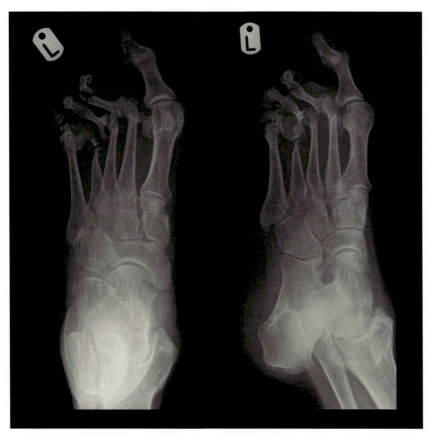

**Figure 9.8** X-ray demonstrating the advanced signs of PsA. © 2022 University Hospitals of North Midlands NHS Trust. All rights reserved.

# Gout

Gout is a form of crystal arthropathy that occurs when crystals of uric acid, in the form of monosodium urate, accumulate on the articular cartilage, tendons and surrounding tissues which provokes an inflammatory response.

Most commonly seen in patients who under-excrete urate due to kidney impairment, or in those who over produce urate such as purine rich diets or increased protein turnover (associated with haematological diseases such as leukaemia or lymphoma). Usually, a clinical diagnosis but X-rays can be used as part of the diagnostic process or to monitor disease progression.

Patients are usually males over the age of 40 with a history of renal impairment; patient may possibly be overweight and taking diuretics. Symptoms usually have a sudden onset (7–10 days) with painful, hot, red and swollen joint. Any joint can be affected; however it is most commonly seen at the MTPJ of the great toe, the midfoot region, the knees and the ankle. Distribution is usually monoarthritic however multiple joints can be affected.

Treatment usually involves NSAIDs for acute attacks. Long-term control includes regulating uric acid production, dietary and alcohol control.

## Radiographic appearance

**Soft-tissue changes:** Caused by the inflammatory response. Soft-tissue enlargement may be visible. The soft tissues may also contain tophi, which are focal soft-tissue densities, sometimes containing calcified deposits.

**Bone erosions:** Persistent inflammation causes damage to the bones' surface resulting in visible erosions. Erosions tend to occur away from the joint margins (para-articular). They often look spherical with a deep, punched-out appearance. Sclerotic edges with overhanging margins = 'rat bite erosions'.

**Secondary signs:** These can include extensive bony destruction due to recurrent episodes. Joint space narrowing and deformity may be present in severe cases but is usually preserved up to this point.

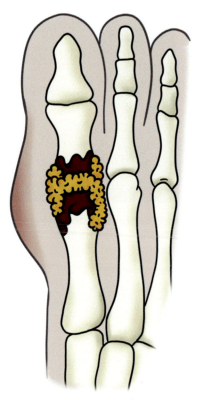

**Figure 9.9** The appearance of crystal deposition at the first MTPJ.

# Osteomyelitis

Osteomyelitis is an inflammation of the bone caused by infection, with *Staphylococcus aureus* being the most common bacteria. Usually a result of haematogenous spread, however, direct infection from open wounds as a result of trauma or surgical procedure or ulceration, typically seen in diabetic patients, is also common.

Infection can occur at any age. However, the location of the infection within the bone can vary with the age of the patient. Adult patients tend to be affected at the epiphysis or subchondral regions of the bone, paediatric patients tend to see the infection within the metaphysis and, in neonatal patients, infection is usually seen in the metaphysis and/or epiphysis. The lower limbs are most affected (especially the toes following nail injury due to the proximity of the periosteum). However, the upper limbs, especially the hands, can be a risk following a biting injury. When the spine is affected, the infection tends to manifest in the lumbar region and the SI joints, with infections in the cervical region being rare.

Patients present with pain, fever and limited movement in the affected area. Bloods will show an elevated erythrocyte sedimentation rate and high white blood cell count.

## Radiographic appearance

**Soft-tissue changes:** Swelling with displacement of the muscle and fat plains and effusions. Gas is seen within the soft tissue due to metabolism of the microorganisms.

**Bony changes:** Regional osteopenia developing into indistinct cortical margins with periosteal reactions and thickening. Over time, bony lysis and bony destruction will occur.

On initial presentation, there may be no radiographic changes and changes caused by osteomyelitis may not be seen on X-ray for 10–14 days in adults, and 5–7 days in children. The affected area must extend at least 1 cm and compromise 30–50% of bone content before being seen on X-ray.

> ## TIP
>
> MRI is the most sensitive and specific modality and considered gold standard. Bone marrow oedema can be seen as early as 1–2 days post-infection and it is good for visualising the soft tissue and joint complications. CT is optimum for visualisation of cortical destruction.

# Septic Arthritis

A destructive arthropathy caused by an intra-articular infection. Can result from direct trauma (including surgery) or spread from infections such as osteomyelitis/cellulitis. Haematogenous spread is the most common cause and the infection can originate in distant sources such as wound infections or pneumonia.

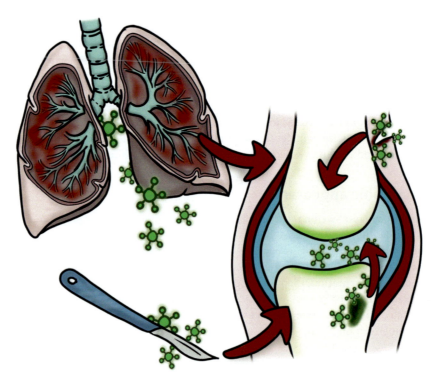

**Figure 9.10** Main sources of septic arthritis.

Usually affects a large joint with an abundant blood supply to the metaphysis such as the knee, hip and shoulder – but any joint can be affected. In paediatric patients the hips are the most commonly affected joint. Hands are susceptible following bite injury and feet can be affected by diabetes. In patients with a history of IVDU the sternoclavicular joints and SIJs are commonly affected.

Patients present with fever/chills and a warm swollen joint with a reduced range of movement. Populations more at risk include those with chronic illness, steroid use, RA, IVDU, end-stage renal disease and joint surgery (including replacements, keyhole and injection). Antibiotics (appropriate for the infecting organism), drainage of the fluid within the joint. If the infection is involving a prosthesis the component needs to be removed (including cement) as anything left in place will act as a point of continued infection. Antibiotic impregnated cement can be used to help resolve the infection and revision of the prosthetic cannot take place until the infection is completely removed, which may require several weeks of treatment.

## Radiographic appearance

X-rays are usually normal at time of presentation. MRI is considered the gold standard in detection and joint aspiration is usually a reliable diagnostic tool.

**Soft-tissue changes:** Earliest changes include swelling, joint effusions and bulging fat plains can sometimes be seen in locations such as the hip (obturator, gluteal and iliopsoas fat pads), the knee (supra=patella effusion or obliteration of Hoffa's fat pad), ankle, shoulder and elbow effusions or wrist effusions (pronator fat pad)

**Bony changes:** Peri-articular osteopenia (demineralisation) caused by hyperaemia. In the early stages, joint space widening may be seen due to the high intra-articular pressure followed by narrowing with erosions. This can be a very rapid process and, in rare cases, can result in ankylosis of the joint. Subluxations can occur due to the surrounding tissue damage.

> ## TIP
>
> Bone on both sides of the joint will be affected – unlike other destructive lesions that tend to only affect one side.

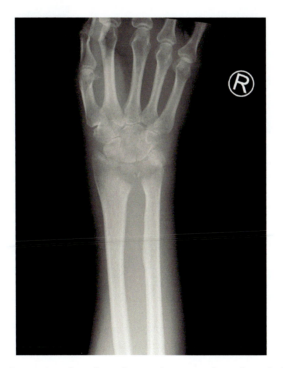

**Figure 9.11** X-ray demonstrating the advanced stages of septic arthritis with soft-tissue swelling and bony destruction on both sides of the joint. © 2022 University Hospitals of North Midlands NHS Trust. All rights reserved.

# Paget's Disease

A chronic bone disorder which is typically seen in the elderly population. It has a classical appearance with prominent, abnormal bone remodelling with a distinctive appearance; bones will appear to increase in size with coarsened trabecular pattern and possible bowing deformities in the long bones and increased kyphosis when seen in the spine. Paget's disease is most commonly seen in the pelvis and spine with the long bones and skull also being affected. It is typically seen affecting multiple bones; however, it can be isolated in some cases. In very rare cases of Paget's, malignant degeneration may occur causing Paget's sarcoma.

The majority of patients will be asymptomatic at time of diagnosis. However, they may present with localised pain and tenderness and reduced range of movement. If the patient is asymptomatic, treatment isn't usually required. However, bisphosphates can be used to help reduce the turnover rate of bone and, if the deformity of the bone is pronounced, surgical procedures such as arthroplasty can be indicated.

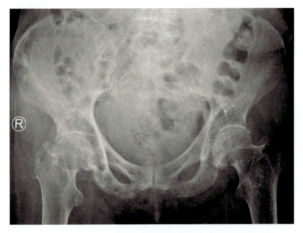

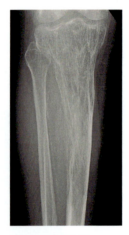

**Figure 9.12** X-ray demonstrating Paget's disease within the pelvis with coarsened trabecular pattern, which is most pronounced in the right inferior and superior pubic rami. © 2022 University Hospitals of North Midlands NHS Trust. All rights reserved.

**Figure 9.13** X-ray demonstrating Paget's disease in the proximal tibia with coarsened trabecular pattern and early bowing deformity. © 2022 University Hospitals of North Midlands NHS Trust. All rights reserved.

## Radiographic appearance

There are three recognised stages of Paget's and radiographic appearance changes within each of these.

**Osteolytic (active) stage:** This stage involves aggressive action of the osteoclasts with resultant bony reabsorption and destruction causing lytic bony lesions with a thinned cortex.

**Mixed stage:** During this stage, the osteoclasts and osteoblasts are working at the same time resulting in a mixture of bone formation and destruction.

**Sclerotic (mixed) stage:** The later stage will demonstrate a mixture of sclerosis and lytic regions within the bone with remodelled, thickened and coarse trabeculae with cortical thinning and bony enlargement with deformity due to bone.

# Chapter 10

# Bone Lesions

## Overview

This chapter will introduce bone lesions, covering both benign and aggressive lesions. We will start with an introduction to the different methods of describing lesions with the aim of understanding which type of lesion we are presented with and help move towards a diagnosis.

We will cover the type of bony changes seen in different lesions as well as their effect on the soft-tissue structures such as the periosteum and the surrounding tissues. Finally, there will be a review of common lytic and sclerotic lesions and their different presentations on X-ray.

## Diagnosis of bone lesions

X-rays can provide information about a number of different factors involved in lesion identification, such as:

- Location of the lesion (anatomical location and the location within the bone)
- Zone of transition
- Type and extent of bone destruction
- Periosteal reaction
- Extent of soft-tissue involvement
- Composition of the lesion (lesion matrix).

A patient's age can also be useful when formulating a diagnosis. Certain lesions are almost exclusively in certain age groups, for example, myeloma, metastatic disease and chondrosarcoma are almost exclusively found in patients over the age of 40, giant cell tumours arise after fusion of the growth plates, whereas chondroblastoma, aneurysmal bone cysts and chondromyoid fibroma are rarely seen in patients over the age of 20.

The number of lesions can also help to differentiate between the various lesions. Primary malignant tumours (such as Ewing's sarcoma, chondrosarcoma, osteosarcoma, fibrosarcoma) don't often present as multiple lesions. If a lesion is multifocal. It usually indicates malignancies such as multiple myeloma, metastatic disease or lymphoma. Multifocal benign lesions include polystotic fibrous dysplasia, Ollier disease, and eosinophilic granuloma.

## Lesion location

A number of lesions have a predilection for specific bones or areas within bones, (e.g. adamantinoma shows a strong preference of the tibia). Sometimes, lesion location alone can help indicate a diagnosis or differential, for example, parosteal osteosarcoma is usually found in the posterior aspect of the distal femur and giant cell tumours are rarely found in any location other than the articular aspect of the bone. The lesion position, in relation to the central axis of the bone, can also help differentiate. Some lesions tend to be centrally located (simple bone cysts, fibrous dysplasia or enchondroma). Other lesions tend to be more eccentrically located (non-ossifying fibroma or aneurysmal bone cyst).

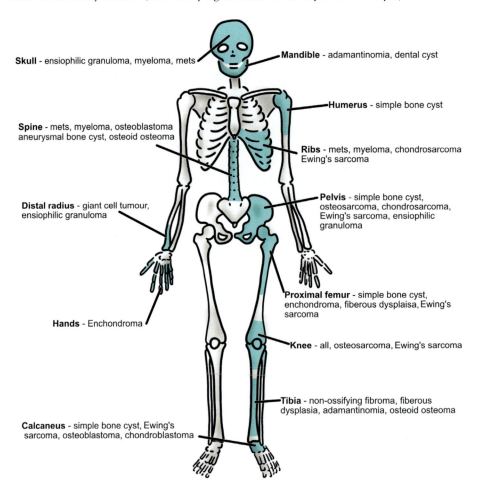

**Skull** - ensiophilic granuloma, myeloma, mets

**Mandible** - adamantinomia, dental cyst

**Humerus** - simple bone cyst

**Spine** - mets, myeloma, osteoblastoma aneurysmal bone cyst, osteoid osteoma

**Ribs** - mets, myeloma, chondrosarcoma Ewing's sarcoma

**Distal radius** - giant cell tumour, ensiophilic granuloma

**Pelvis** - simple bone cyst, osteosarcoma, chondrosarcoma, Ewing's sarcoma, ensiophilic granuloma

**Proximal femur** - simple bone cyst, enchondroma, fiberous dysplaisa, Ewing's sarcoma

**Hands** - Enchondroma

**Knee** - all, osteosarcoma, Ewing's sarcoma

**Tibia** - non-ossifying fibroma, fiberous dysplasia, adamantinomia, osteoid osteoma

**Calcaneus** - simple bone cyst, Ewing's sarcoma, osteoblastoma, chondroblastoma

**Figure 10.1** The typical locations of bone lesions.

## Zone of transition

The borders of a lesion can help to reveal how fast the lesion is growing, which gives an insight into how aggressive the lesion may be. Well-defined borders indicate a slow-growing lesion, which has a greater chance of being benign. Ill-defined borders indicate a faster growing lesion, with a higher chance of being aggressive or malignant.

Margins can be divided into three broad categories.

1. Sharply demarcated with a sclerotic border.
2. Sharply demarcated without sclerosis.
3. Ill-defined.

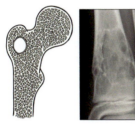

**Figure 10.2** An illustration and X-ray demonstrating a sharply demarcated lesion with a sclerotic border. © 2022 University Hospitals of North Midlands NHS Trust. All rights reserved.

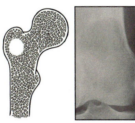

**Figure 10.3** An illustration and X-ray demonstrating a sharply demarcated lesion without a sclerotic border. © 2022 University Hospitals of North Midlands NHS Trust. All rights reserved.

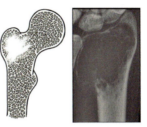

**Figure 10.4** An illustration and X-ray demonstrating an ill-defined lesion. © 2022 University Hospitals of North Midlands NHS Trust. All rights reserved.

## Type of bone destruction

Bony destruction can be caused by two main processes: the effect of the actual tumour cells on the bone or by the normal action of the osteoclasts reacting to abnormal growth of the tumour.

Trabecular (cancellous) bone is destroyed at a quicker rate than cortical bone, however, cortical bone loss can be seen earlier on plain film imaging (as its density is very homogenous). Approximately 70% of cortical bone must be lost before it is visible on plain film imaging.

There are three main types of bone destruction:

1. **Geographic destruction:** Uniform bone loss with sharply outline borders.
2. **'Moth eaten' destruction:** Characterized by multiple, small lytic areas – often clustered together.
3. **Permeative destruction:** Small ovoid lucencies or lucent streaks that are not ill defined.

Bone destruction alone cannot define specific lesions. However, it is helpful in differentiating between benign and malignant lesions, for example, benign, slow-growing lesions tend to show geographical destruction, aggressive faster-growing lesions show either moth-eaten or permeative destruction patterns. It should be noted that some non-malignant (but aggressive) lesions may demonstrate aggressive destruction patterns.

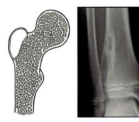
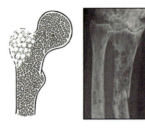
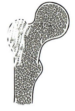
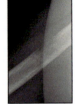

**Figure 10.5** Illustration and X-ray demonstrating geographical bony destruction. © 2022 University Hospitals of North Midlands NHS Trust. All rights reserved.

**Figure 10.6** Illustration and X-ray demonstrating moth-eaten bony destruction. © 2022 University Hospitals of North Midlands NHS Trust. All rights reserved.

**Figure 10.7** Illustration and X-ray demonstrating permeative bone destruction. © 2022 University Hospitals of North Midlands NHS Trust. All rights reserved.

## Periosteal reaction

A periosteal reaction is a non-specific response to an irritation of the bone. This irritation can be caused by a number of factors such as trauma, infection or bone lesions. Periosteal reactions can be classified as non-aggressive (benign) or aggressive and can be described according to the pattern of the reaction.

### Aggressive reactions

- Interrupted or discontinuous.
- Associated with fast-growing and aggressive processes. These processes can include malignancies such as osteosarcoma, Ewing's sarcoma, etc. However, an aggressive reaction does not always indicate a malignancy and can be caused by a benign (but with an aggressive appearance) process such as osteomyelitis.
- Types include laminated (onion skin), speculated (sunburst/hair on end), disorganised, Codman's triangle.

### Non-aggressive (benign) reactions

- Uninterrupted or continuous.
- Tend to be associated with slow-growing underlying process. The slow growth gives the periosteum more time to lay down new bone (however, this new bone tends not to be as dense as the cortical bone).
- Solid reaction (thick or thin).
- Thick irregular reaction.
- Can also be called 'cortical thickening'.
- Can be associated with fracture callus formation or slow-growing lesions, such as osteoid osteoma.

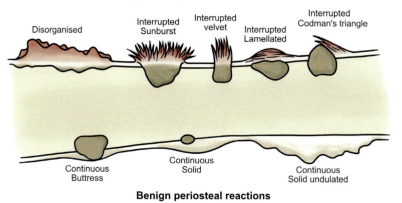

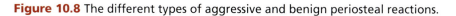

**Aggressive periosteal reactions**

Disorganised

Interrupted
Sunburst

Interrupted
velvet

Interrupted
Lamellated

Interrupted
Codman's triangle

Continuous
Buttress

Continuous
Solid

Continuous
Solid undulated

**Benign periosteal reactions**

**Figure 10.8** The different types of aggressive and benign periosteal reactions.

## Soft-tissue involvement

Presence of a soft-tissue mass is a reliable indicator of an aggressive process. It is important to determine if soft-tissue involvement is an extension of a primary bone tumour or, if it is a primary soft-tissue tumour involving the bone. Primary malignant bone tumours usually cause a periosteal reaction when they break the cortex.

## Lesion matrix

When discussing the matrix of a lesion, you are describing the type of tissue that makes up the lesion, for example, is the lesion made up of chondroid, fibrous, osteoid or adipose tissues? Mineralisation of the lesion is the description of the calcification of the matrix.

Lesions can be described as lytic, sclerotic or mixed, e.g. simple bone cysts and giant cell tumours are lytic lesions, enostosis (bone islands) are sclerotic lesions and adamantinomas are mixed lesions.

Mineralisation patterns can be used to suggest a differential diagnosis. For example, chondral lesions often produce punctate, flocculent or rings and arc-type mineralisation (seen in enchondromas, chondrosarcoma, chondroblastoma, etc.). Bone-forming lesions often have a fluffy, amorphous, cloud-like mineralisation, which looks opaque on X-ray images (seen in osteosarcoma).

## TIP

Describe lesions as benign or aggressive – Do not use the word malignant when describing lesions – it is important to remember that not all aggressive lesions are malignant. Some highly aggressive lesions (such as bone/joint infection) have no malignant process involved.

# FEGNOMASHIC

FEGNOMASHIC is a mnemonic for the differential diagnosis of lucent/lytic bone lesions. This is not an exhaustive list but covers the most commonly seen lytic lesions (95%). Most bone lesions present as osteolytic lesions so it is important to have a good understanding of the range of differentials.

- Fibrous dysplasia
- Enchondroma
- Eosinophilic granuloma
- Giant Cell tumour
- Non-ossifying fibroma
- Osteoblastoma
- Mets
- Myeloma
- Aneurysmal bone cyst
- Simple/solitary bone cyst
- Hyperthyroidism
- Infection
- Chondroblastoma
- Chondromyxoid fibroma.

## Fibrous dysplasia

A benign bone lesion caused by the replacement of the medullary bone with fibrous tissues. Commonly seen in 3–15-year-olds and is typically asymptomatic unless fractured. Due to the remodelling of the bone it is weaker, so is prone to fracture.

X-ray appearance:

- Endosteal scalloping (reabsorption of the inner cortical layer)
- Cortical thinning
- No periosteal reaction
- Ground-glass appearance to the matrix
- Well-defined lesions
- When in long bones, may cause bowing deformity (Shepherd's crook appearance within the proximal femur)
- Common locations for the lesion include the pelvis, femur, ribs, skull/jaw (if in the tibia consider adamantinoma – a malignant tumour with a similar appearance).

CT is the best modality for demonstrating the fibrous matrix and can be used to confirm diagnosis. Biopsy is not required for diagnosis. Treatment isn't usually required; however, the affected bones may require stabilisation due to weakness or treatment following fracture.

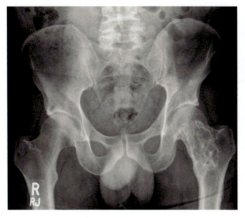

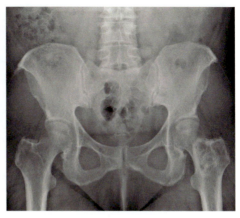

**Figure 10.9** AP pelvic X-ray demonstrating a large fibrous dysplasia within the left proximal femur. © 2022 University Hospitals of North Midlands NHS Trust. All rights reserved.

**Figure 10.10** AP pelvic X-ray demonstrating a fibrous dysplasia within the left proximal femur. © 2022 University Hospitals of North Midlands NHS Trust. All rights reserved.

## Enchondroma

A benign cartilaginous tumour commonly seen in younger patients (10–30 years old). Usually asymptomatic and an incidental finding, pain and swelling can occur with malignant degeneration or a pathological fracture. The lesion is prone to fracture to the thinned and weakened bone.

X-ray appearance:

- Well-defined, lytic lesion (when in the small bones of the hands and feet) and slightly expansile. When in the long bones, enchondromas appear as a well-defined sclerotic chondroid calcification (when seen in the long bones, consider bony infarct as a differential).
- May have endosteal scalloping.
- No periosteal reaction.
- Rarely in the epiphysis (if seen in the epiphysis, consider chondrosarcoma as a differential).
- **Common locations:** Small bones of the hands and feet. Less commonly seen in the femur, tibia and humerus.

Treatment is not usually required.

- **Ollier disease (enchondromatosis):** Multiple enchondromas usually affecting the hands and feet.
- **Maffucci syndrome:** Multiple enchondromas with associated haemangioma.

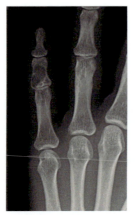

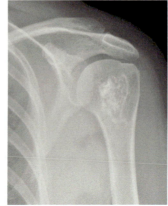

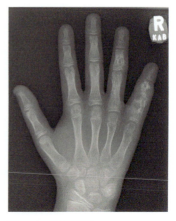

**Figure 10.11** X-ray demonstrating an enchondroma in the middle phalanx of the fifth finger. © 2022 University Hospitals of North Midlands NHS Trust. All rights reserved.

**Figure 10.12** X-ray demonstrating an enchondroma in the proximal humerus. © 2022 University Hospitals of North Midlands NHS Trust. All rights reserved.

**Figure 10.13** X-ray demonstrating Ollier disease in the phalanxes of the fourth and fifth fingers. © 2022 University Hospitals of North Midlands NHS Trust. All rights reserved.

## Eosinophilic granuloma

A benign solitary tumour which is commonly seen in older children and young adults. Patients typically present with pain, swelling and tenderness at the lesion. However, it can be asymptomatic in some cases.

X-ray appearance:

- Various presentations depending on region affected
- **Skull:** Punched-out lytic lesion with no sclerotic rim
- **Mandible:** Irregular lucent regions involving the alveolar bone (floating tooth sign)
- **Spine:** Vertebral plana (most common cause of plana in children)
- **Long bones:** Depending upon disease phase. Permeative and aggressive appearance, endosteal scalloping and cortical thinning, periosteal reaction, soft-tissue mass
- **Common locations:** Skull (most common), pelvis, femur, humerus, ribs, mandible, spine and ribs.

Treatment includes excision and curettage with chemo/radiotherapy. Most lesions will spontaneously resolve over 1–2 years. Excellent prognosis if confined to the skeleton.

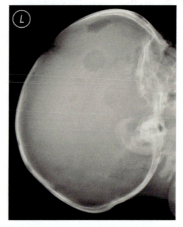

**Figure 10.14** X-ray demonstrating eosinophilic granuloma with a punched-out lesion within the skull of a paediatric patient. © 2022 University Hospitals of North Midlands NHS Trust. All rights reserved.

# Giant cell tumour

A radiographically aggressive lesion seen in the mature skeleton. The patient's growth plates must be fused for a GCT to form. GCTs are usually benign, however, malignant degeneration can occur in very rare cases. Patients' presentations can include pain, soft-tissue mass and impingement on adjacent structures.

X-ray appearance:

- **Growth plates must be closed**
- Expansile – may be very large at diagnosis
- Well-defined with no sclerotic rim
- Abuts the articular surface
- No periosteal reaction (unless fractured)
- Eccentric
- **Common locations:** Knee (most common), wrist, sacrum, vertebral bodies.

Treatment includes curettage with packing (bone chips or polymethylmethacrylate) with radiotherapy.

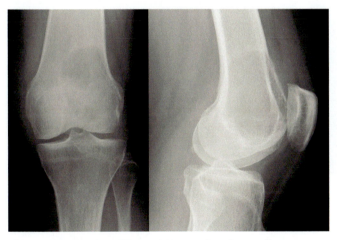

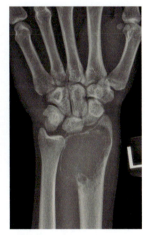

**Figure 10.15** AP and lateral X-ray of a giant cell tumour within with lateral condyle of a left femur. © 2022 University Hospitals of North Midlands NHS Trust. All rights reserved.

**Figure 10.16** DP X-ray of a giant cell tumour within the distal radius. The lesion shows poor definition of the proximal aspect suggestive of malignant degeneration. © 2022 University Hospitals of North Midlands NHS Trust. All rights reserved.

## Non-ossifying fibroma

Benign fibrous tumour also known as a fibrous cortical defect when smaller than 2 cm. Usually seen in children and young adults but can be seen in older patients, they spontaneously resolve and ossify with age. Typically, an incidental finding with no associated pain.

X-ray appearance:

- Well-defined, multiloculated lucent lesion, usually with a sclerotic rim
- Typically, in the metaphysis emanating from the cortex
- Eccentric and slightly expansile
- No periosteal reaction
- As they ossify, they will become sclerotic until disappearing
- **Common locations:** Tibia is the most common location but can be seen in the upper extremities.

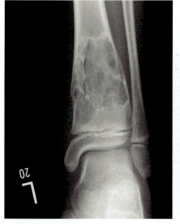 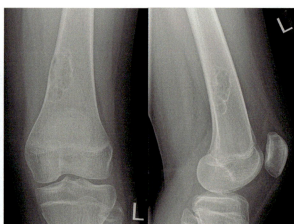

**Figure 10.17** AP X-ray demonstrating a large non-ossifying fibroma in the distal left tibia. © 2022 University Hospitals of North Midlands NHS Trust. All rights reserved.

**Figure 10.18** AP and lateral X-ray demonstrating a non-ossifying fibroma abutting the medial cortex of the distal left femur. © 2022 University Hospitals of North Midlands NHS Trust. All rights reserved.

## Osteoblastoma

A rare benign bone forming tumour usually seen in 10–30-year-olds. Presents with pain, worse at night with minimal response to salicylates (aspirin).

X-ray appearance:

- Lytic lesion with a rim of sclerosis
- Usually larger than 2 cm, otherwise, it resembles an osteoid osteoma. However osteoid osteomas do not grow and respond well to NSAIDs
- Tend to be expansile, sometimes with cortical destruction
- Internal calcification is sometimes present
- Consider osteoblastoma when an aneurysmal bone cyst is a differential
- **Common locations:** Spine (posterior column), long bones (metaphysis or distal diaphysis).

Treatment includes surgical management with excision. The lesion is very vascular so prone to intraoperative bleeding.

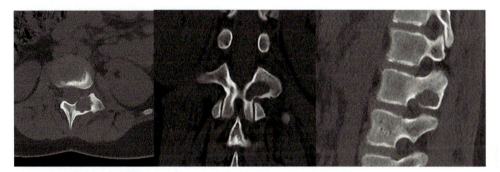

**Figure 10.19** Axial, coronal and sagittal CT views of an osteoblastoma within the pedicle of L2. © 2022 University Hospitals of North Midlands NHS Trust. All rights reserved.

## Metastatic disease

Malignant lesions are secondary to a primary sarcoma. Metastatic disease accounts for the majority of all malignant bone tumours. In all patients over 40 years old, metastases (mets) should be considered for any lytic lesions whether they appear benign or aggressive radiologically. Metastatic disease is usually pre-diagnosed and is typically asymptomatic, however, the lesion weakens the bone making it prone to fracture.

X-ray appearance:

- Can have mixed appearances – lytic, sclerotic, or mixed.
- Can be focal, diffuse or expansile.
- Difficult to identify on X-ray. There must be 30–50% bone mineral loss before they can be seen on X-ray. MRI is the gold standard for identification of mets.
- **Common locations:** Spine, pelvis, skull, proximal femurs and humerus.

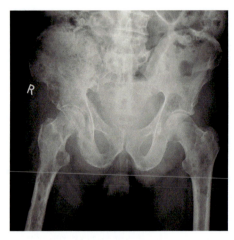

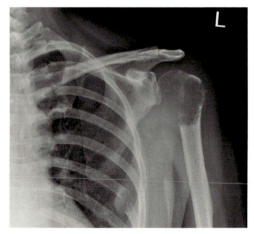

**Figure 10.20** AP pelvic X-ray demonstrating multiple destructive lucent metastatic deposits within the pelvis and proximal femur. © 2022 University Hospitals of North Midlands NHS Trust. All rights reserved.

**Figure 10.21** AP shoulder X-ray demonstrating a large lucent metastatic deposit within the left proximal humerus, with a further lucent metastatic deposit within the 7th posterior rib with a pathological rib fracture. © 2022 University Hospitals of North Midlands NHS Trust. All rights reserved.

## Myeloma

Malignancy of the bone marrow, typically seen in patients over 40 years of age (and should be considered as a differential for any lytic lesion in the over 40-year-old population until excluded). Patients present with pain which is exacerbated on activity, anaemia, renal failure, proteinuria and hypercalcemia.

X-ray appearance:

- Numerous well-circumscribed lytic bone lesions
- Punched-out lucencies (raindrop skull)
- Endosteal scalloping
- Generalised osteopenia
- **Common locations:** Vertebral bodies are the most commonly affected followed by the ribs, skull, shoulder, pelvis, long bones. MRI is more sensitive for the detection of multiple lesions.

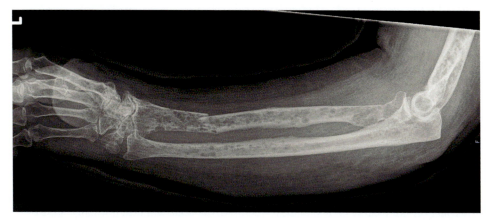

**Figure 10.22** AP X-ray of a left radius and ulna demonstrating the multiple punched-out lucencies of multiple myeloma, with a pathological fracture of the radius. © 2022 University Hospitals of North Midlands NHS Trust. All rights reserved.

## Aneurysmal bone cyst

Benign blood-filled tumour of variable sizes. Primarily seen in children and adolescents and patients may present with pain, which can be sudden onset if fractured, a palpable lump and restricted movement.

X-ray appearance:

- Sharply defined with thin sclerotic margins
- Expansile
- Eccentric within the metaphysis, adjacent to unfused growth plate
- **Common locations:** long bones, lower limb including proximal tibia and fibula and femur. Also seen in the spine and sacrum and the craniofacial region.

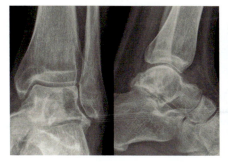

**Figure 10.23** AP and lateral ankle X-ray demonstrating an aneurysmal bone cyst within body of the left talus. © 2022 University Hospitals of North Midlands NHS Trust. All rights reserved.

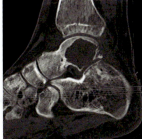

**Figure 10.24** Sagittal CT view demonstrating an aneurysmal bone cyst within body of the left talus. © 2022 University Hospitals of North Midlands NHS Trust. All rights reserved.

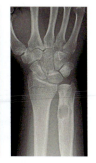

**Figure 10.25** DP wrist X-ray demonstrating an aneurysmal bone cyst within the left ulna. © 2022 University Hospitals of North Midlands NHS Trust. All rights reserved.

## Simple bone cyst

A benign bone lesion filled with a clear fluid, typically seen in younger patients but rarely seen over the age of 30. Asymptomatic unless fractured and prone to fracture due to the thinned weakened bone.

X-ray appearance:

- Well-defined lytic lesions with a narrow zone of transition.
- May demonstrate an expansile appearance with cortical thinning.
- When fractured, may present with a 'fallen fragment' sign which is pathognomonic for a simple bone cyst.
- **Common locations:** Proximal humerus, proximal femur and long bones. Rarely seen in adults, but they are found in unusual locations such as the talus, calcaneum and ilium.

Treatment is not usually necessary as, if fractured, the bone will heal normally. Sometimes surgical curettage and grafting may be required.

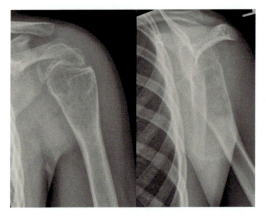

**Figure 10.26** AP and lateral humerus X-ray demonstrating a simple bone cyst within the proximal left humerus.

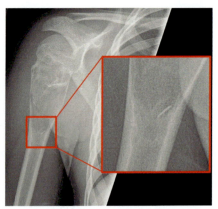

**Figure 10.27** X-ray demonstrating a pathological fracture through a simple bone cyst. Note the fallen fragment within the distal aspect of the bone cyst. © 2022 University Hospitals of North Midlands NHS Trust. All rights reserved.

## Hyperthyroidism (Brown's tumour)

This is a bone lesion caused by excessive osteoclast activity related to hyperparathyroidism.

X-ray appearance:

- Patients must have other signs of hyperparathyroidism.
- Wide range of appearances similar to a giant cell tumour.
- Sometimes expansile with cortical thinning.
- Well-defined, lytic lesion, little reactive bone, and the cortex may be thinned and expansile.
- **Common locations:** Mandible, ribs, clavicle and pelvis.

When hyperparathyroidism is treated, the tumour will undergo sclerosis and eventually vanish.

## Infection

Infection/osteomyelitis can mimic bone lesions and appear as a radiographically aggressive process which can be found across a range of age groups.

X-ray appearance:

- Must be larger than 1 cm and compromise 30–50% of bone mineral content to be seen on X-ray.
- Early findings may take 5–7 days to be seen in children and 10–14 days in adults on X-ray. MRI is much more sensitive and considered the gold standard.
- Earliest sign can be effusions.
- Osteopenia with bony lysis.
- Endosteal scalloping and cortical loss.
- Aggressive periosteal reactions.
- Gas within the soft tissues.
- **Common locations:** No typical location, however, the lower limb is the most commonly affected, with infections of the hands and spine also frequently seen.

Treatment involves intravenous antibiotics, drainage and debridement. Amputation may be required if medical treatment fails or if there is a risk to life.

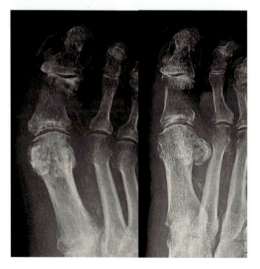

**Figure 10.28** DP and oblique X-ray of a right great toe demonstrating osteomyelitis. Gas is seen within the distal soft tissues with bony erosions and destruction. © 2022 University Hospitals of North Midlands NHS Trust. All rights reserved.

## Chondroblastoma

A benign lesion almost exclusively seen in patients under the age of 30. Non-specific presentation; joint pain, tenderness, swelling, muscle wasting, mass.

X-ray appearance:

- Only occurs in the epiphysis
- Geographic lytic lesions with a sclerotic margin
- Eccentric

- May have endosteal scalloping or epiphysis cortical expansion
- May extend adjacent to the epiphysis when expanding
- **Common locations:** Epiphysis of long bones (femur, tibia and humerus) or within apophysis (greater trochanter, greater tuberosity, acromion, calcaneum and talus).

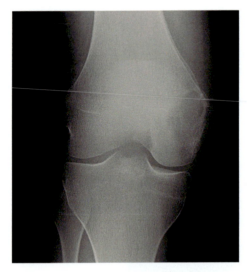

**Figure 10.29** AP X-ray demonstrating a chondroblastoma within the medial condyle of a right femur. © 2022 University Hospitals of North Midlands NHS Trust. All rights reserved.

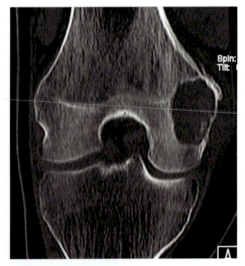

**Figure 10.30** Coronal CT view of a chondroblastoma within the medial condyle of a right femur. © 2022 University Hospitals of North Midlands NHS Trust. All rights reserved.

## Chondromyxoid fibroma

Extremely rare, but benign lesion most commonly seen before the age of 30. Patients present with pain, swelling and restricted range of movement in the affected limb.

X-ray appearance:

- Resembles a non-ossifying fibroma
- Well-defined expansile lytic lesion with a sclerotic margin
- Geographical bone destruction
- No periosteal reaction
- **Common locations:** Metaphyseal region of long bones, with the upper third of the tibia being the most common site. Small bones of the foot, distal femur, pelvis and sacrum are also affected.

# Sclerotic Bone Lesions

Sclerotic bone lesions can be differentiated according to the patients age. Some of the more commonly seen lesions include enostosis, bony infarcts, osteoid osteoma and osteochondroma. Some of the previously described lytic lesions may also have a sclerotic appearance (such as fibrous dysplasia or mets).

## Enostosis (bone island)

A common benign sclerotic bone lesion, typically asymptomatic and usually an incidental finding.

X-ray appearance:

- Small round or oval foci of dense sclerotic bone
- Can demonstrate feathered or brush-like margins
- Typically, less than 1 cm in size. However, larger bone islands can be seen (usually in the pelvis) – anything greater than 2 cm is considered a giant bone island
- **Common locations:** Can occur anywhere within the skeleton, but most commonly seen in the pelvis, long bone and ribs
- **Osteopoikilosis:** multiple benign enostosis. Develops during childhood and does not regress; it can be seen in all age groups.

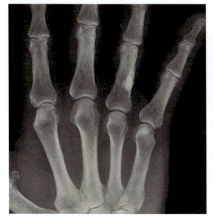

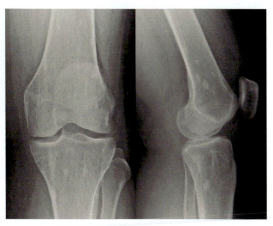

**Figure 10.31** DP right hand X-ray demonstrating a large solitary enostosis within the proximal phalanx of the fourth finger. © 2022 University Hospitals of North Midlands NHS Trust. All rights reserved.

**Figure 10.32** AP and lateral X-ray of a left knee demonstrating osteopoikilosis (multiple enostosis) throughout the distal femur and proximal tibial. © 2022 University Hospitals of North Midlands NHS Trust. All rights reserved.

## Osteoid osteoma

A benign bone forming tumour, usually found in children (occasionally adolescents). Patients present with night pain, which is relieved with salicylate analgesia (aspirin).

X-ray appearance:

- Small lucent nidus (less than 1.5–2 cm) – usually round or oval
- Nidus is surrounded by a rim of reactive sclerosis
- May be a reduction in bone density – caused by disuse due to pain
- Cortical thickening
- **Common locations:** Seen in long bones, but any bone can be affected. Most commonly seen in the femoral neck, mid-tibial diaphysis, phalanges and vertebra (lumbar most common)
- CT is the gold standard for diagnosis – demonstrates the nidus most effectively.

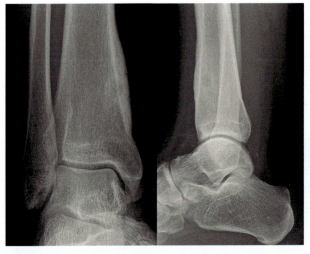 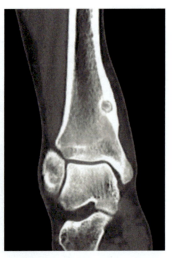

**Figure 10.33** AP and lateral X-ray of a right ankle demonstrating an osteoid osteoma in the medial cortex of the distal tibia – the nidus can be seen as a subtle lucency within the cortical thickening. © 2022 University Hospitals of North Midlands NHS Trust. All rights reserved.

**Figure 10.34** Coronal CT view of an osteoid osteoma in the medial cortex of the distal tibia. © 2022 University Hospitals of North Midlands NHS Trust. All rights reserved.

## Bone infarct

Osteonecrosis within the metaphysis and diaphysis of the long bones (osteonecrosis within the epiphysis is classified as avascular necrosis). Caused by interrupted blood supply to the bone and is linked to trauma, alcoholism, pancreatitis, sickle-cell disease, corticosteroid excess and radiotherapy.

X-ray appearance:

- Similar appearance to an enchondroma within long bones
- Intermedullary calcification within the metaphysis or diaphysis
- Commonly seen with a shell-like calcification surrounding the infarct (this is not seen in enchondromas).

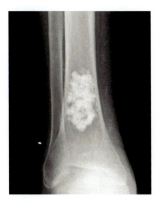

**Figure 10.35** X-ray demonstrating a bony infarct within the distal tibia. © 2022 University Hospitals of North Midlands NHS Trust. All rights reserved.

## Osteochondroma (bony exostosis)

A common benign sclerotic bone lesion. There is cartilage capped projection of bone. Malignant degeneration of the cartilage cap is possible but rare. Asymptomatic and usually an incidental finding. However, if painful, should be assessed for irritation/impingement of surrounding structures, fracture of the neck of the osteochondroma or malignant degeneration.

X-ray appearance:

- Sessile or pedunculated
- Metaphyseal region projection away from the epiphysis
- Can be a range of sizes
- Cartilage capped – the cartilage component is not seen on X-ray. However, some caps may demonstrate calcifications. Thick caps (more than 1 cm) should be considered for malignant degeneration
- Malignant degeneration should be considered when:
  - there is growth of the osteochondroma after skeletal maturity
  - the cortex becomes indistinct
  - erosion or destruction of adjacent bone
  - if there is development of an adjacent soft-tissue mass or irregular soft-tissue calcifications
- **Common locations:** Lower limb (distal femur is the most common, tibia) and humerus
- **Multiple hereditary exostoses (osteochondromatosis):** Development of multiple osteochondromas. Radiographic appearance is exactly the same as solitary osteochondromas. Malignant degeneration is more common.

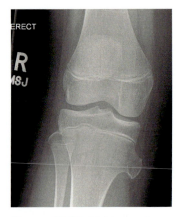

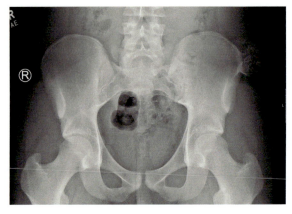

**Figure 10.36** AP X-ray of a right knee demonstrating an osteochondroma projecting from the medial cortex of the proximal tibia. © 2022 University Hospitals of North Midlands NHS Trust. All rights reserved.

**Figure 10.37** AP pelvic X-ray demonstrating a large osteochondroma projecting from the left iliac crest. © 2022 University Hospitals of North Midlands NHS Trust. All rights reserved.

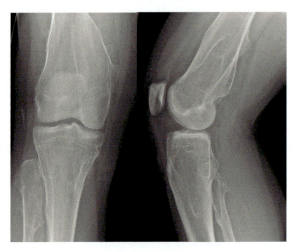

**Figure 10.38** AP and lateral X-ray of a right knee demonstrating multiple osteochondromas in the distal femur, proximal tibia and proximal fibula. © 2022 University Hospitals of North Midlands NHS Trust. All rights reserved.

## Subungual exostosis

A benign osteocartilagenous tumour that forms below the nail bed. Commonly seen in children and young adolescents. Presents with pain and swelling with possible ulcer formation.

X-ray appearance:

- Bony projection from the dorsal surface of the distal phalanx
- Usually connected to the underlying bone
- Well-circumscribed, however may be difficult to differentiate from the medulla and cortex
- **Common locations:** Under the nail bed. Most commonly seen at the first toe.

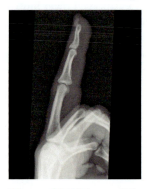

**Figure 10.39** Lateral X-ray of a third finger demonstrating a subungual exostosis. © 2022 University Hospitals of North Midlands NHS Trust. All rights reserved.

## Sclerotic metastatic disease

Malignant lesions secondary to a primary sarcoma, these commonly originate from prostate or breast primary lesions. However, breast metastatic deposits will initially present as lytic lesions before turning sclerotic after chemotherapy. Less commonly associated with lung, lymphoma or carcinoid primary. Must be included as a differential for any sclerotic lesions in patients over 40 years old.

**Common locations:** Vertebra, pelvic, skull, proximal femur and humerus.

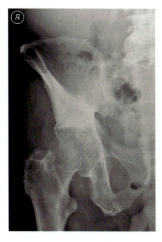

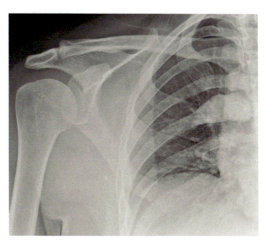

**Figure 10.40** AP X-ray of a right hip demonstrating a large sclerotic metastatic deposit within the right ilium. © 2022 University Hospitals of North Midlands NHS Trust. All rights reserved.

**Figure 10.41** AP right shoulder X-ray demonstrating a sclerotic expansile met within the posterior aspect of the sixth rib. © 2022 University Hospitals of North Midlands NHS Trust. All rights reserved.

## Osteosarcoma

A malignant primary bone tumour. There are several categories and subcategories of osteosarcoma. Often presents with pain and occasionally an associated soft-tissue mass or swelling. In some cases, there may be no symptoms and patients may only present following a pathological fracture.

A primary osteosarcoma is idiopathic and not associated with other malignancies and disease processes. It typically occurs in younger patients, with most cases occurring before the age of 20 due to active bone growth.

Primary osteosarcomas are further subtyped:

- **Conventional:** Intramedullary.
- **Small cell:** Metaphyseal region of long bones. Permeative and lytic involving the medulla.
- **Telangiectatic:** Metaphysis of long bone, expansile and lytic containing multiple fluid levels.

- **Low-grade central:** Usually affects older patients 19–54 years. Affects the medulla of the metaphysis (usually the tibia or fibula). Expansile and destructive septal trabecular or sclerotic appearance.
- **Surface osteosarcoma:** Parosteal surface osteosarcomas arise from the outer layer of the periosteum and are the most common type of surface osteosarcoma. Periosteal surface osteosarcomas arise from the inner layer of the periosteum with demonstrated perpendicular periosteal reaction. High-grade surface osteosarcomas are very rare, arising from the outer cortex of the bone and encases the circumference of the bone.

Secondary osteosarcomas are associated with other pre-existing conditions; usually secondary to malignant degeneration of Paget's disease, extensive bony infarcts or post-radiotherapy.

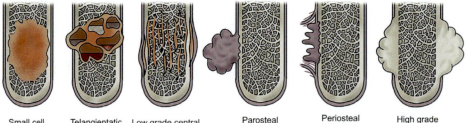

Small cell    Telangientatic   Low grade central    Parosteal    Periosteal    High grade

**Figure 10.42** Illustration demonstrating the subtypes of primary osteosarcoma.

## Radiographic appearance

- Medullary and cortical bone destruction
- Wide zone of transition with a permeative or motheaten appearance
- **Aggressive periosteal reaction:** Characteristic sunburst appearance. Lifting of the periosteum leading to Codman's triangle. A lamellated (onion skin) reaction is less commonly seen
- **Soft-tissue mass:** New bone formation within the soft tissues
- Matrix appearance can be variable depending on the tumour bone production with an ill-defined, fluffy or cloud-like matrix.

Plain film is useful for initial diagnosis. MRI can then be used to assess the extension of the tumour and soft-tissue involvement. CT and bone scans are used to assess for metastatic deposit and staging.

## Distribution

Primary lesions tend to occur at the long bones:

- Femur (especially distally) most common
- Tibia (especially proximally)
- Humerus.

Also seen at other sites such as the fibula, mandible, maxilla and vertebra. However, these are seen less commonly. Secondary lesions can be seen throughout the body, usually following the distribution pattern of the underlying condition that cause them.

## Treatment

Involves surgical resection (usually amputation) followed by chemotherapy. If there is the possibility of saving the affected limb, it is possible to treat with chemotherapy to reduce tumour size, bone resection and prosthesis insertion.

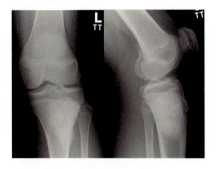

**Figure 10.43** AP and lateral X-ray of a left knee demonstrating an osteosarcoma within the proximal tibia. © 2022 University Hospitals of North Midlands NHS Trust. All rights reserved.

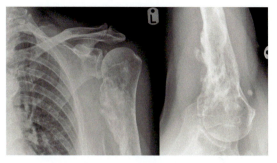

**Figure 10.44** AP and axial X-ray of a left shoulder demonstrating an osteosarcoma within the proximal humerus. © 2022 University Hospitals of North Midlands NHS Trust. All rights reserved.

# Ewing's Sarcoma

Malignant primary bone tumour of childhood, typically occurring in patients between the ages of 5 and 25 years. Patients often present with limited range of movement with pain and a palpable soft-tissue mass. Blood tests will show a raised ESR.

## Radiographic appearance

- Variable appearance – but will demonstrate aggressive features
- Common findings include a large lesion with a moth-eaten or permeative appearance with a wide zone of transition
- Aggressive periosteal reactions such as lamellated (onion skin) or spiculated appearances are often seen
- Cortical destruction is often seen
- Lesion may appear sclerotic in some cases
- Associated soft-tissue mass is a common finding
- Less commonly seen features include cortical thickening, bony remodelling and soft-tissue calcifications.

## Distribution

Most lesions occurring in long bones are nearly always within the metadiaphyseal or diaphyseal regions. They are typically seen arising from the medullary bone with wide skeletal distribution, but most common in the lower limb. The femur is the most common, followed by pelvis, upper limb and spine/ribs.

## Treatment

Chemotherapy with radiotherapy and surgical resection should be considered depending on lesion location and size.

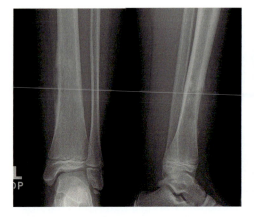

**Figure 10.45** AP and lateral X-ray of a left ankle demonstrating Ewing's sarcoma within the medial cortex of the distal tibia. © 2022 University Hospitals of North Midlands NHS Trust. All rights reserved.

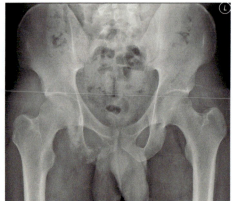

**Figure 10.46** AP pelvic X-ray of Ewing's sarcoma at the right inferior pubic rami. © 2022 University Hospitals of North Midlands NHS Trust. All rights reserved.

# Chondrosarcoma

Malignant cartilaginous tumours, usually affecting patient between the ages of 30 and 70 years. Patients typically present with pain, swelling and mass.

Can be characterised as primary or secondary chondrosarcoma. Primary chondrosarcomas arise de novo, with secondary chondrosarcoma arising from malignant transformation of benign bone lesion, such as osteochondromas or enchondromas.

## Radiographic appearance

- Can have a range of appearances
- Usually a large mass; most are larger than 4 cm at diagnosis
- Usually lytic with a moth-eaten or permeative appearance
- Endosteal scalloping, cortical thickening or remodelling with associated periosteal reactions
- Calcification within the lesion, usually in a ring and arcs pattern or a 'popcorn' pattern.

## Distribution

Most common sites include the pelvis, proximal femur and humerus. Seen less commonly in the spine, scapular, sternum, head and neck and the facial region. Chondrosarcomas within the hand and feet are rare and are usually the result of malignant transformation of enchondromas.

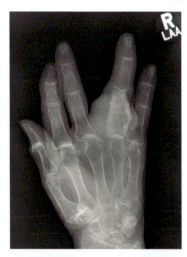

**Figure 10.47** DP hand X-ray demonstrating a secondary chondrosarcoma in the proximal phalanx of the fourth finger, following malignant transformation of an enchondroma. © 2022 University Hospitals of North Midlands NHS Trust. All rights reserved.

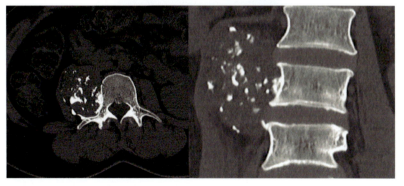

**Figure 10.48** Axial and sagittal CT views demonstrating a chondrosarcoma which is at the level of L2, clearly showing the ring and arcs pattern of the lesion calcification. © 2022 University Hospitals of North Midlands NHS Trust. All rights reserved.

## TIP

Do not forget to use the FEGNOMASHIC mnemonic when reviewing bone lesions.

# Index